TIPPING THE SCALES

Ethical and Legal Dilemmas in Managing Severe Eating Disorders

TIPPING THE SCALES

Ethical and Legal Dilemmas in Managing Severe Eating Disorders

Edited by

Patricia Westmoreland, M.D.

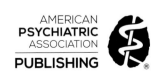

AMERICAN
PSYCHIATRIC
ASSOCIATION
PUBLISHING

Copyright © 2021 American Psychiatric Association Publishing

ALL RIGHTS RESERVED

First Edition

Manufactured in the United States of America on acid-free paper
25   24   23   22   21   5   4   3   2   1

American Psychiatric Association Publishing
800 Maine Avenue SW, Suite 900
Washington, DC 20024-2812
www.appi.org

Library of Congress Cataloging-in-Publication Data
Names: Westmoreland, Patricia, editor. | American Psychiatric Association
    Publishing, issuing body.
Title: Tipping the scales : ethical and legal dilemmas in managing severe eating
    disorders / edited by Patricia Westmoreland.
Other titles: Tipping the scales (Westmoreland)
Description: First edition. | Washington, DC : American Psychiatric Association
    Publishing, [2021] | Includes bibliographical references and index.
Identifiers: LCCN 2020040579 (print) | LCCN 2020040580 (ebook) | ISBN
    9781615373499 (paperback ; alk. paper) | ISBN 9781615373772 (ebook)
Subjects: MESH: Anorexia Nervosa—therapy | Psychiatry—ethics | Psychiatry—
    legislation & jurisprudence | Bulimia Nervosa—therapy | Feeding and Eating
    Disorders of Childhood—therapy
Classification: LCC RC552.A5 (print) | LCC RC552.A5 (ebook) | NLM WM 175
| DDC 616.85/26206—dc23
LC record available at https://lccn.loc.gov/2020040579
LC ebook record available at https://lccn.loc.gov/2020040580

British Library Cataloguing in Publication Data
A CIP record is available from the British Library.

For Bob, Matthew and Carys, and our four legged friends:

"The world is truly round and seems to start and end with those we love."

—*Nelson Mandela*

Contents

Philip S. Mehler, M.D.

Russell Marx, M.D.

Ken Weiner, M.D.

1 Treatment of Eating Disorders:

Michael Spaulding-Barclay, M.D., M.S.

Arnold Andersen, M.D.

Joel Yager, M.D.

2

Kaila Rudolph, M.D., M.P.H., M.B.E.

Rebecca Weintraub Brendel, M.D., J.D.

3

Angela S. Guarda, M.D.

Colleen C. Schreyer, Ph.D.

Contributors

Arnold Andersen, M.D.
Professor Emeritus, Department of Psychiatry, University of Iowa College of Medicine, Iowa City, Iowa

Ovidio Bermudez, M.D., FAAP, FSAHM, FAED, Fiaedp, C.E.D.S.
Clinical Professor of Pediatrics and Psychiatry, University of Colorado School of Medicine, Eating Recovery Center, Denver, Colorado

Leah Brar, M.D.
Attending Psychiatrist, Medical Center of Aurora; Assistant Professor of Psychiatry, Rocky Vista University, Aurora, Colorado

Wayne Bowers, Ph.D.
Professor, Department of Psychiatry, Roy and Lucille Carver College of Medicine, University of Iowa, Iowa City, Iowa

Rebecca Weintraub Brendel, M.D., J.D.
Director, Master of Bioethics Degree Program; Associate Director, Center for Bioethics; Assistant Professor of Psychiatry, Harvard Medical School, Boston, Massachusetts

Isis Elzakkers, M.D., Ph.D.
Formerly with Altrecht Eating Disorders Rintveld, Altrecht Mental Health Institute, Utrecht, The Netherlands

Libby Erickson, D.O.
Attending Psychiatrist, Eating Recovery Center, Denver, Colorado

Cynthia M.A. Geppert, M.D., M.A., M.P.H., M.B.E., D.P.S., M.S.J, FACLP, DFAPA, FASAM, HEC-C
Ethics Consultant, VA National Center for Ethics in Health Care, Washington, DC; Chief Consultation Psychiatry, New Mexico VA Health Care System; Professor of Psychiatry and Internal Medicine and Director of Ethics Education, University of New Mexico School of Medicine, Albuquerque, New Mexico; Adjunct Professor of Bioethics, Alden March Bioethics Institute, Albany Medical College, Albany, New York

Dennis Gibson, M.D.
Associate Professor, Department of Internal Medicine, University of Colorado; Assistant Medical Director, ACUTE at Denver Health, Denver, Colorado

Angela S. Guarda, M.D.
Stephen and Jean Robinson Associate Professor of Psychiatry and Behavioral Sciences and Director, Johns Hopkins Eating Disorders Program, Johns Hopkins School of Medicine, Baltimore, Maryland

Annette Hanson, M.D.
Clinical Assistant Professor and Director, Forensic Psychiatry Fellowship, University of Maryland, Clifton T. Perkins Hospital, Jessup, Maryland

Phillipa Hay, M.D.
Professor and Foundation Chair of Mental Health, Translational Health Research Institute, Western Sydney University School of Medicine, Penrith, New South Wales, Australia

Jeanne Kerwin, D.M.H., HEC-C
Consultant in Bioethics and Palliative Care, Atlantic Health System, Morristown; Faculty, Drew University, Medical Humanities Graduate Program, Madison, New Jersey

Barbara Kessel, D.O.
Attending Psychiatrist, Eating Recovery Center, Denver, Colorado

Mark Komrad, M.D.
Clinical Assistant Professor of Psychiatry, University of Maryland, College Park, Maryland; Clinical Assistant Professor of Psychiatry, Tulane University, New Orleans, Louisiana; Instructor in Psychiatry, Johns Hopkins University, Baltimore, Maryland

Cushla McKinney, Ph.D., M.B.H.L.
Research Fellow, Department of Pathology, Dunedin School of Medicine, University of Otago, Dunedin, New Zealand

Russell Marx, M.D.
Associate Professor of Psychiatry, University of Colorado; Attending Psychiatrist, ACUTE at Denver Health, Denver, Colorado

Philip S. Mehler, M.D.
Glassman Professor of Internal Medicine, University of Colorado; Founder and Executive Medical Director, ACUTE at Denver Health; President and Chief Science Officer, Eating Recovery Center, Denver, Colorado

Anne-Marie O'Melia, M.D.
Chief Medical Officer, Eating Recovery Center, Denver, Colorado

Kaila Rudolph, M.D., M.P.H., M.B.E.
Attending Consultation Liaison Psychiatrist, Boston Medical Center; Instructor of Psychiatry, Boston University School of Medicine, Boston, Massachusetts

Colleen C. Schreyer, Ph.D.
Assistant Professor of Psychiatry and Behavioral Sciences, Johns Hopkins School of Medicine, Baltimore, Maryland

Michael Spaulding-Barclay, M.D., M.S.
Medical Director, Child and Adolescent Services, Eating Recovery Center, Denver, Colorado

Michael Stafford, J.D.
City and County Attorney, Denver County, Denver, Colorado

Stephen Touyz, Ph.D.
Professor Emeritus, School of Psychology and Inside Out Institute, Boden Collaboration, Charles Perkins Centre, University of Sydney 2006, New South Wales, Australia

Elizabeth Wassenaar, M.D.
Medical Director, Eating Recovery Center, Denver, Colorado

Ken Weiner, M.D.
Founder and former CEO, Eating Recovery Center, Denver, Colorado

Patricia Westmoreland, M.D.
Forensic Psychiatrist and Consultant, ACUTE at Denver Health; Adjunct Assistant Professor of Psychiatry, University of Colorado, Denver, Colorado

Joel Yager, M.D.
Professor, Department of Psychiatry, Anschutz Medical Campus, Aurora, Colorado

Introduction

Philip S. Mehler, M.D.
Russell Marx, M.D.
Ken Weiner, M.D.

Morbidity and Mortality Associated With Eating Disorders

In contrast to patients with other mental health disorders, such as schizophrenia or bipolar illness, for whom a medical physician rarely needs to be involved in care delivery, patients with eating disorders (EDs) have a litany of significant medical complications that demand close oversight by a medical doctor knowledgeable in treating these disorders. However, prior to the 1980s, little available literature elucidated the best medical practices for patients with EDs, and currently, very few physicians have much medical expertise in this specialized area. This is disconcerting, because these patients are known to be frequent utilizers of the medical system who are often admitted to hospitals and emergency departments for medical complications of their disorders (Dooley-Hash et al. 2019). In addition, anorexia nervosa (AN) has the highest mortality rate of any mental disorder except opioid abuse (Chesney et al. 2014), and the standardized mortality ratio for bulimia nervosa (BN) is almost twice that seen in age-matched control subjects (Kask et al. 2016). Moreover, much of the excessive mortality rate in AN is attributable to medical complications. Thus, there is an impelling need for this book, which highlights the medicolegal and ethical challenges in treating individuals with EDs.

While reading this book, keep in mind the medical complexities inherent in caring for individuals with EDs. These patients are known to have a multitude of gastrointestinal abdominal complaints. The real challenge is in ferreting out functionally based from organically based symptoms due to the weight loss and malnutrition that characterize AN or the purging behaviors of BN. In AN, restricting type, symptoms of fullness, bloating, and early satiety are common due to gastroparesis, which almost universally develops as weight loss becomes more severe (Norris et al. 2016). However, a critical gap in our knowledge exists as to the percent of ideal body weight (%IBW) below which gastroparesis develops and the weight that must be attained for gastroparesis to resolve. Similarly, superior mesenteric artery syndrome is increasingly recognized as a cause of upper abdominal pain that develops in patients with AN soon after they commence eating. Again, we do not know the %IBW below which the syndrome develops or at which it resolves. These are critically important organic conditions to recognize, because their ongoing and undiagnosed presence can markedly impede successful refeeding and weight restoration. Another common gastrointestinal medical dilemma involves abnormal elevations in liver enzymes (aspartate transaminase and alanine aminotransferase) seen in patients with AN. Very few potential causes for their elevation have been identified, including malnutrition and death of the liver cells versus exuberant refeeding and deposition of carbohydrates and fat in the liver. The treatment of these two conditions is diametrically opposed; the former is treated through ongoing aggressive weight restoration and the latter with a possible reduction in calories or at least a change in the macro composition of the diet. No clear surrogates exist to predict which cause is most likely and how best to intervene (Rosen et al. 2017).

Furthermore, as previously noted, mortality is very high in AN. Sudden cardiac death has been proposed to be an important etiological reason for this; however, the exact cause of sudden cardiac death in AN remains enigmatic. The once-posited mechanism of a prolonged QTc interval causing torsades de pointes and ventricular tachycardia is no longer in vogue. Excessive QT dispersion or lack of heart rate variability along with cardiac fibrosis and increased global longitudinal strain are currently areas of intense research in the quest to attenuate the risk of cardiac demise more effectively in patients with AN (Sachs et al. 2015).

Another important area lacking definitive medical evidence is the optimal way to treat the dangerous and highly prevalent loss of bone mineral density found in patients with AN (Garber et al. 2015). Although no medicinally based approaches were in use prior to the late 1990s, in the past 20 years, a number of different medicines with potential benefit have been found to both slow loss of bone mineral density and improve it. No head-to-head comparative trial or randomized controlled trial (RCT) has yet been performed to guide optimal treatment of this common and devastating complication, which has long-term adverse consequences, including fragility fractures and chronic pain.

Moreover, notwithstanding the irrefutably critical role of nutrition in achieving sustained recovery in AN, evidenced-based RCTs to guide the optimal refeeding of these patients do not exist. Although progressive oral feeding is the basic tenet of weight restoration, in the range of 3–4 lb/week for an inpatient-residential level of care, many permutations on this theme exist, including continuous nasogastric or nasojejunal feedings, nocturnal enteral feedings, or combinations of oral plus supplemental enteral continuous or bolus feedings. All of these approaches have support in the literature (Golden and Mehler 2020), and all may be relevant for patients with AN. Yet, despite nutrition being such an essential part of recovery, in the end, this field cannot currently opine the best route to pursue. However, it is clear that the process and rate of weight restoration have evolved over the past decade to espouse more aggressive escalation of delivered calories and the rate of expected weight gain per week to avoid "underfeeding." New interest has developed in the recently described concept of "weight disruption," and treatment teams are cautioned to focus not only on absolute %IBW but also on the rapidity and delta change in the patient's weight loss as part of the body image distortions of EDs (Golden and Mehler 2020).

Finally, one important and relevant medical gap in knowledge exists regarding the entity known as Pseudo-Bartter syndrome (PBS). This syndrome, which involves complex electrolyte and acid-base aberrations and a proclivity toward severely distressing and rapid edema formation in patients who abruptly cease purging behaviors, has been increasingly recognized as a factor that may interfere with successfully treating BN (Bahia et al. 2012). Part of the reason for its ongoing adverse impact is the gap in knowledge as to how best to prevent PBS and to treat it safely when it does occur. This lack of a definitive approach is, in part, a root cause of the treatment conundrum for these patients and why they may require multiple attempts to treat their BN. No current data indicate which type of purging behavior is associated with the greatest risk of PBS.

Part of the uniqueness of EDs, in contrast to other mental health disorders, is the intricate interplay between their medical and psychiatric manifestations. The hope is that ongoing focus on and deliberation about these disorders will lead to increased recognition of this interaction, which in turn will exhort ongoing research into the effective ways to prevent and treat the ubiquitous medical comorbidity that is inextricably tied to a successful outcome for these patients.

This is a much-needed book because progress in the medical and psychological treatment of EDs over the past half-century has shown us what we *can* do but sometimes leaves unanswered questions about what we *should* do in difficult situations, such as the case of a person with a severe and enduring eating disorder (SEED) who is symptomatic, resists treatment, and requires repeated involuntary hospitalizations. This book explores the ethical and legal dimensions of these difficult questions. Recent presentations at Academy of Eating Disorders meetings have had such titles as "What's the Right Call? Ethical Considerations in Compulsory Treatment of Eating Disorders" and "Anorexia Nervosa, Limits of Capacity and Futility." How can the study of ethics be helpful in looking at these questions?

Origin of Ethics

The word *ethics* derives from the Greek word *ethos*, which relates to our ideals about character and value. Aristotle noted that the subject of ethics was "good action," with its principal concern being the nature of human well-being, and recommended that we study ethics to improve our lives. However, he was clear that "ethical theory does not offer a decision procedure" because "what must be done in any particular occasion by a virtuous agent depends on the circumstances, and these vary so much from one occasion to another that there is no possibility of stating a series of rules, however complicated, that collectively solve every practical problem" (Kraut 2018). The Hebrew approach to ethics has both similarities and differences. Jewish law, the Halakha, provides "an elaborate, highly detailed scale of values that establishes orders of priorities in a great variety of cases and situations" (Steinsaltz 1999, p. 49). A one-sentence summary of this body of law was given by the great sage Hillel: "What you hate to have done unto you, do not do to others" (quoted in Steinsaltz 1999, p. 48). However, as noted Talmudic scholar Adin Steinsaltz (1999) has written,

> We tend to expect moral laws to give clear answers, but in fact, attempts to formulate moral universals are inherently incomplete. Broad-spectrum definitions of good do not provide black-and-white, yes-or-no answers. In most cases the choices we face are between shades of gray, namely between a lesser good and a greater good, a lesser evil and a greater evil. (p. 48)

If ethical theory cannot offer a decision procedure, what value *can* it offer? First, it can help clarify thinking. According to Aristotle, "practical reasoning always presupposes that one has some end, some goal one is trying to achieve; and the task of reasoning is to determine how that goal is to be accomplished." Regarding identifying a goal, he noted, "Virtue makes the goal right, practical wisdom the things leading to it" (Kraut 2018). How do we arrive at the proper notion of virtue in a situation such as that of a patient with SEED who refuses treatment? The multiple competing values in this example may not be compatible with each other. For example, saving a life is a core value of medicine, and EDs have an exceedingly high mortality rate. On the other hand, relief of suffering is also a core value of medicine, and refeeding can bring about both physical and emotional discomfort in these patients. Patient autonomy is also an important value and brings up the question of who gets to set the goals of treatment. Parties with an investment in this outcome include the patient, family, caregivers, health care systems, and society at large. Important components of goal determination involve the patient's age, the length of illness, the adequacy of prior treatments, and the patient's capacity. *Capacity* requires that patients be able to understand information about their condition, reason through the information needed to make decisions, appreciate the consequences of those decisions, and communicate their decisions.

Role of Ethics in Compelling Treatment for Patients With SEEDs

Hillel's dictum—"what you hate to have done onto you, do not do to others"—may require modification in the case of a patient with SEED who faces potential involuntary treatment based on evaluation of his or her capacity. Judicial decisions about competence to refuse ED treatment show wide variance depending on the state, province, or country in which one resides. Judgments regarding "mental soundness" may also vary at different points in a person's illness. This book explains the basic principles of ethics and addresses the concept of capacity and the role of involuntary treatment for patients with EDs. The historically problematic concept of "futility" of treatment is also discussed (see Chapter 11, "Futility"). No good evidence base yet exists for predicting the possibility of treating an individual patient successfully. Treatments are constantly evolving, and no patients have yet failed all of the possible combinations of potentially successful treatments. Emerging treatments that are generating interest include transcranial magnetic stimulation, deep brain stimulation, and ketamine, as described in Chapter 8 ("Novel Treatments for Patients With Severe and Enduring Eating Disorders"). Some of the most promising areas of new research involve the role of the gastrointestinal system in the construction of feelings and mood. Given the obvious importance of the gastrointestinal system in the process of eating, research on the influences of the microbiome in anxiety and depression may discover new treatments for individuals with SEEDs whose prognosis has been called "futile." Perception of futility in the treatment of these challenging cases may reflect burnout of the treatment team rather than unlikelihood of success. This may also contribute to the emergence in Europe of physician-assisted death and euthanasia in this population, discussed in Chapter 12 ("Eating Disorders and Physician-Assisted Death").

Challenges in the Treatment of Patients With SEEDs

Resource Allocation

Clarification of values is helpful not only for individual practitioners and treatment teams but also for larger health care systems. Some issues raised about the ethics of continued involuntary treatment of people with SEEDs involve "resource constraint" and the futility of further treatment. One of the values most closely associated with classical ethical theory is that of justice. Is it *just* to expend vast quantities of resources for patients with cancer or rare genetic illnesses but to plead resource constraint when denying life-saving treatment to patients with SEED? In some European countries, people with chronic psychiatric and medical illnesses (of which an ED is both) are increasingly being pressured to consider physician-assisted suicide or euthanasia to avoid becoming a burden to society, as explained in Chapter 12. This may, in truth, have more to do with the stigma of psychiatric illness than with fairness for patients with EDs. We are building better health care systems for cancer and other diseases—why not for EDs? Famed economist Michael Porter (2006) described "the virtuous circle in health care delivery" (p. 161). This might be a good model for the future evolution of treatment of patients with SEEDs within larger health care systems. The hope is that this investment in recovery will yield not only greater success but also a greater sense of hope and purpose among practitioners that will be transmitted to their challenging yet deserving patients and families.

Construction of Specialized Facilities

Chapter 1 ("Treatment of Eating Disorders") discusses in more detail the evolution of ED treatment centers, but it is worth mentioning how this intersected in one center with the evolution of involuntary treatment in its resident state. In 2008, Drs. Ken Weiner and Emmett Bishop founded the Eating Recovery Center (ERC), with the intention of creating a mission-driven company. Their mission was to provide the best care for people with EDs, their families, and their referring health care professionals. They envisioned a fully integrated health care system for the 30%–40% of patients who either could not recover with a good multidisciplinary outpatient team or did not have access to such outpatient expertise in their area.

Rising Need for Involuntary Treatment

When ERC opened October 21, 2008, the intent was to help patients with moderate, severe, and extreme forms of ED. As such, a subset of patients who were the "sickest of the sick" were frequently admitted. Unfortunately, these patients were ambivalent about entering treatment, and as we began treating and feeding them, many signed out. This was bad for patients, terrifying for families, and discouraging for staff, who had become attached to their patients and cared deeply about them. Insurance companies were also unhappy, because they had made a financial commitment to care and gotten nothing tangible for their investment. In 2010, ERC petitioned the state of Colorado and, after considerable dialogue, was granted the ability to provide involuntary treatment in 24-hour, partial hospitalization, intensive outpatient, and outpatient programs. As reflected in Chapter 3 ("Coercion in Treatment"), feedback from patients who had felt coerced into treatment showed that most found it helpful (Guarda et al. 2007). They recognized that the illness had hijacked their brain and that they had been incapable of making a good decision at the time. ERC's commitment to caring for those with the most extreme forms of ED has also led to changes in case law around certification, as detailed in Chapter 6, "Civil Commitment."

ERC has also taken an individualized approach to dealing with futility in patients with and staff treating SEEDs. Depending on the patient's age, treatment history, and support system, the treatment team will either "go to the mat" to achieve full recovery or engage in a harm reduction model. At times, patients have left treatment requesting palliative care, and several chapters in this book explain the difference between *harm reduction* (Chapter 9) and *palliative care* (Chapter 10) and how palliative care differs from *futility* (Chapter 11).

Finally, although we recognize that treatment is sometimes futile, this book discusses the difference between allowing SEEDs to *cause* an person's demise and offering physician-assisted death or euthanasia, options that are currently not available in the United States and have been deemed unethical by the World Medical Association, American Medical Association, and American Psychiatric Association. We hope that expounding on the medicolegal and ethical complexities of ED treatment will help physicians and mental health professionals (as well as patients) make the best decisions for healing and recovery or, if this is neither possible nor desired, for dignified passage within the bounds of current knowledge and the ethics of palliative end-of-life care.

References

Bahia A, Mascolo M, Gaudiani JL, Mehler PS: PseudoBartter syndrome in eating disorders. Int J Eat Disord 45(1):150–153, 2012

Chesney E, Goodwin GM, Fazel S: Risks of all-cause and suicide mortality in mental disorders: a meta-review. World Psychiatry 13(2):153–160, 2014

Dooley-Hash S, Adams M, Walton MA, et al: The prevalence and correlates of eating disorders in adult emergency department patients. Int J Eat Disord 52:1281–1290, 2019

Garber AK, Sawyer SM, Golden NH, et al: A systematic review of approaches to refeeding in patients with anorexia nervosa. Int J Eat Disord 49:293–310, 2015

Golden NH, Mehler PS: Atypical anorexia nervosa can be just as bad. Cleve Clin J Med 87(3):172–174, 2020

Guarda AS, Pinto AM, Coughlin JW, et al: Perceived coercion and change in perceived need for admission in patients hospitalized for eating disorders. Am J Psychiatry 164(1):108–114, 2007

Kask J, Ekselius L, Brandt L, et al: Mortality in women with anorexia nervosa: the role of comorbid psychiatric disorders. Psychosom Med 78:910–919, 2016

Kraut R: Aristotle's ethics, in The Stanford Encyclopedia of Philosophy, Summer 2018 Edition. Edited by Zalta EN. Stanford, CA, Center for the Study of Language and Information, Stanford University, 2018

Norris ML, Harrison ME, Isserlin L, et al: Gastrointestinal complications associated with anorexia nervosa: a systematic review. Int J Eat Disord 49:216–237, 2016

Porter M: Redefining Health Care. Boston, MA, Harvard Business School Press, 2006

Rosen E, Bakshi N, Watters A, et al: Hepatic complications of anorexia nervosa. Dig Dis Sci 62(11):2977–2981, 2017

Sachs KV, Harnke B, Mehler PS, Krantz MJ: Cardiovascular complications of anorexia nervosa: a systematic review. Int J Eat Disord 49:238–248, 2015

Steinsaltz A: Simple Words. New York, Simon and Schuster, 1999

1

Treatment of Eating Disorders

An Historical Perspective

Michael Spaulding-Barclay, M.D., M.S.
Arnold Andersen, M.D.
Joel Yager, M.D.

Eating Disorders as Sociocultural Phenomena Versus Serious Medical Illnesses

Food-related preoccupations and concerns about body weight and shape have forever been part of society. People with sensitive or extreme temperaments sometimes become zealously preoccupied with prominent cultural attitudes and practices, such as those pertaining to feasting, fasting, food-related taboos and rituals, and concerns with weight and shape. At times, these individuals are ineffective at coping with these concerns and begin to behave maladaptively, consequently falling into states of psychological and physiological impairment (i.e., disorders). For these susceptible outliers, sociocultural pressures and fads may funnel their personal vulnerabilities into the shape of eating disorders (EDs).

Before examining the sociocultural phenomena that give EDs form, we must first consider what makes people susceptible to them. Three studies are illustrative. The first evaluated childhood obsessive-compulsive personality traits and found that childhood perfectionism and inflexibility (rigidity) were particularly strong predictors of ED, as well as being rule-bound, displaying doubt and cautiousness, and having a drive for order and symmetry. This was more pronounced for anorexia nervosa (AN) than for bulimia nervosa (BN). Each trait increased the additional risk of developing an ED by an approximate factor of seven (Anderluh et al. 2003). The second study identified childhood anxiety symptoms at age 10. The authors linked physical anxiety symptoms to the development of BN and linked worrying to the development of AN during adolescence (Schaumberg et al. 2019). A third study identified several concurrent risk factors for BN, necessitating the presence of both general psychiatric vulnerabilities and specific factors concerning attitudes and behaviors about weight and dieting. People who developed mood, anxiety, and substance use disorders were found to have increased likelihood of personal vulnerabilities (e.g., childhood characteristics, premorbid psychiatric disorders, behavioral problems, lifetime parental psychiatric disorders) and environmental factors (e.g., parental problems, disruptive events, parental caring and involvement patterns, recent parental psychiatric disorders, teasing or bullying, and sexual or physical abuse). Histories of childhood abuse and parental alcoholism were particularly common. In addition to these general psychiatric vulnerabilities (which usually result in depression), young women who developed BN had higher rates of environmental risk factors such as dieting, obesity, and parental ED (Fairburn et al. 1997).

These and other studies suggest that when vulnerable individuals who tend to be obsessional, perfectionistic, moody, and anxious are exposed to cultural attitudes and values that stress feasting, fasting, food taboos and rituals, and preoccupations with weight and shape, some embody and transmute these sociocultural phenomena into serious EDs.

Feasting

In the beginning of human existence, some food was available, but often not enough. Food scarcities may have driven evolutionary pressures toward the appearance of "thrifty genes" that offered easier storage of body fat during plentiful times as insurance against lean times, thus fostering overweight and obesity during periods of abundance. Festive gorging might have occurred after successful large game hunts, or at harvest times once agriculture developed. Experts have pondered the significance and meaning of the prehistoric "Venus of Willendorf" carving (dated to approximately 28,000–

25,000 B.C.E.), but it seems probable that this portly feminine figure with huge, pendulous breasts was a figure of adoration and admiration rather than scorn. After societies evolved from egalitarian sharing to rich and poor strata, the rich developed fancy banquets; in Ancient Rome, they went so far as to institute vomitoria for participants who overgorged, thus architecturally supporting and culturally condoning purging behavior.

With contemporary food abundances in developed areas, rates of obesity and, correspondingly one may assume, of binge eating disorder (BED), are increasing. Pima Indians (the Othama or Akimel O'odham people) in Southern Arizona have a great deal more significant obesity and diabetes mellitus than their counterparts in northern Mexico, just across the border, whose livelihoods require considerably more daily caloric expenditure. In the "supersize" culture of fast foods and oversized portions that is promulgated in the United States and has been exported to the rest of the world, rates of obesity have grown significantly.

Fasting

Variously but widely practiced in many cultures and religions, intentional fasts devotionally demonstrate self-denial and may produce altered states of consciousness. Fasts are practiced in Baha'i, Eastern Orthodox Christianity, Evangelical Christianity, Hinduism, Islam, Jainism, Judaism, Native American religions, Roman Catholicism, and Taoism. Moses, Jesus, and Buddha were all said to have engaged in prolonged fasts associated with their spiritual pursuits.

Historically, dating from the fifth century B.C.E. in India, the Jain religious practice of *Sallekhana* involves voluntarily fasting to death by gradually reducing one's intake of food and liquids, representing the thinning of human passions and the body. Chandragupta Maurya (340–297 B.C.E.), who founded the historically significant Mauryan Empire, is said to have renounced his throne to spend several years following his Jain guru and to have died by self-starvation. Large populations, including entire families, followed his example. A takeaway lesson here is that high-profile, influential leaders who adopt dramatic eating practices often become trendsetters and lead others to devotionally or blindly follow, even to the followers' significant detriment.

Extreme versions of fasting and self-denial have clearly generated near-epidemic, clinically significant fashion trends. In *anorexia mirabilis*, during the fourteenth and fifteenth centuries, women intending to demonstrate Christian devotion through self-denial became obsessed with mortification of the body and abhorrent of the flesh. In parallel with some cases of contemporary AN, religious fasting in these women triggered extreme and persistent self-denial of food. Many achieved altered states of consciousness, often experienced as ecstatic "highs." The more spiritually perfectionistic and single-minded among them starved themselves and died in large numbers (Espi Forcen and Espi Forcen 2015). The Roman Catholic Church canonized several hundred of these women as saints, the most prominent among them St. Catherine of Siena. Clinical descriptions of these women in "holy anorexia" suggest strong resemblances to contemporary descriptions of AN.

Food-Related Taboos and Rituals

Taboos and rituals concerning food and eating are extremely common and ancient across societies. Mosaic laws of *kashruth* (defining kosher foods, animal slaughter, and food preparation, such as prohibiting pork and shellfish) date to more than a millennium B.C.E. Certain Jain, Buddhist, and Hindu traditions advocating nonviolence to all living things and associated taboos on eating beef and requirements of strict vegetarianism, particularly among the Brahmin class, date to at least 500 B.C.E. Some anthropologists argue that such taboos originated in economic considerations or for health reasons, whereas others believe food taboos usefully set kinship groups apart from one another, differences that defined marital options. Strictly observant Brahmins and Jains abstain from onions and garlic as well (perhaps reflecting allium sensitivities on the part of some ancient thought leaders).

Regardless of their origins, millions of people accept food taboos "off the shelf," developing deep disgust and fear of certain foods and feelings of shame and guilt over related transgressions. In contemporary society, subgroups with food aversions are increasingly common (e.g., vegan, gluten-free, sugar-abstinent, various allergies). Clearly, rule-following individuals with obsessional and compulsive tendencies might be particularly prone to adopt food rules involving food elimination, portion-size limitations, and so on, growing rules on top of rules, to the point of caloric and micronutrient deficiencies associated with avoidant/restrictive food intake disorder (ARFID), orthorexia nervosa, or AN.

Preoccupations With Weight and Shape

For both sexes, physical appearances denoting attractiveness and health have been associated with higher social status and preferential mate selection for virtually all of recorded history. Throughout the ages, artists have depicted what different epochs and ethnicities variously considered most desirable. Over the past two centuries, we can easily trace fads and fashions showing strong influences of high-status opinion leaders on weight- and shape-related practices. The following are a few salient illustrations.

In the mid-nineteenth century, Princess Elizabeth of Austria, Queen of Hungary (1837–1898; peak influence circa 1859–1860), who was then one of the highest-status women in Europe, helped set the stage for widespread dieting, corseting, and "tight-wasting" among young women of royal connection and persuasion. Known to binge-eat and purge, she weighed herself obsessively multiple times daily; throughout her adult life, her weight varied from BMIs of 14–17. Numerous princesses followed her lead, and high-status young females started to show clinical symptoms that culminated in the original independent descriptions of AN among upper-class women by Gull in England and Lasègue in France (Gull 1873; Lasègue 1873).

Certain technologies became more widespread and might have also increased attention to shape and weight. Although crude mirrors were available beforehand, the first silver-glass mirror was invented in 1835, and the general availability of household mirrors developed in the mid- to late nineteenth century. Similarly, street-corner "penny scales" first became popular in the 1920s and 1930s ("measure your weight for a penny"), and affordable household bathroom scales first became widely available in the 1940s. Just as internet and cellphone addictions required the invention and widespread availability of those technologies, mirrors and scales permitted easier obsessional and compulsive attention to weight and shape.

Starting in the late nineteenth century and blossoming in the twentieth, trickle-down influences on shape and weight also became much more pronounced with modern advertising and mass media. One of the first fads to widely promote slender female body shapes, the "flapper" fashions of the 1920s, was accompanied by increased reporting in college newspapers of purging behaviors among college women. This trend abated in the 1930s, 1940s, and 1950s, during which time curvaceous body shapes among high-status and celebrity women became more prominent.

However, during the 1960s, several mass culture influences converged to promote the social desirability of slender appearance in high-status (predominantly white) women. Along with the sexual revolution, Helen Gurley Brown, editor-in-chief and top-tier trendsetter at *Cosmopolitan* magazine, pushed images of slim fashion models, lauding the thin look. Among celebrities, slim American and British actresses and models became top fashion icons. In contrast to previous, somewhat older, and more solidly built presidential wives, Jacqueline Kennedy cut a slim, youthful figure. The advent of early television and the appearance of many actresses as heavier on screen than they were in real life may have led some actresses to slim down to improve their on-screen appearance. George Balanchine, the most prominent

American ballet director, favored increasingly thin dancers who were much thinner than their European counterparts, and Hugh Hefner, publisher of *Playboy* magazine, chose slimmer women in the 1960s and 1970s to personify female sexuality as "Playmate" centerfolds.

As popular culture became stocked with growing numbers of fashion magazines portraying unrealistically slim, airbrushed fashion models, many women became obsessed with these magazines, and those vulnerable to EDs consistently found themselves feeling worse after reading them. Television fashion shows flourished that featured predominantly slim models (as currently represented by shows such as *Project Runway* and *America's Next Top Model*). When first exposed to slim feminine Western images on television, well-built Polynesian Island teenage females who had been content with themselves previously became increasingly self-conscious and dissatisfied with their appearance and for the first time ever began to develop EDs. In post-apartheid South Africa, Westernization may be impacting attitudes toward shape and weight, resulting in greater likelihood of EDs (Morris and Szabo 2013). Similar shifts have been seen in Latina/Hispanic populations, leading some authorities to view EDs not only as culture bound syndromes but also as markers of cultural change (Miller and Pumariega 2001).

Today, adding to the ubiquitous sniping, competitive, gossipy, and snarky "friendships" that add to normative adolescent peer pressures, youth are contending with powerful social media sites, such as Facebook, Instagram, and Snapchat, that are dominated by visual images and afford further opportunities for negative self-evaluation by appearance-preoccupied, insecure, self-doubting, anxious young women who strongly link self-esteem to physical appearance. As these young women find their own appearances to be wanting and inferior, they appear more vulnerable to developing EDs.

Evolution of ED Treatment Programs

The treatment of any disorder depends upon several factors: 1) contemporaneous general theories of illness (e.g., Hippocratic-Galenic theory of the four humors); 2) specific concepts of etiology for the disorder (psychosocial, neurochemical, psychodynamic); 3) the diagnostic criteria and terminology in use (*anorexia nervosa* vs. *pubertätsmagersucht* vs. *hysterical anorexia*); and 4) the training methods of treating clinicians. Challenges to whatever treatment methods are currently in vogue lead to a period of defensive (and often angry) skepticism about the need for change and to replacement by a new method (paradigm shift). Physicians once believed that peptic ulcers were caused by excess acid production in the stomach from either stress or dietary indiscretion, and thus they prescribed antacids, low-acid foods, and acid-buffering medications. Only after Warren and Marshall, using heroic methods of self-inoculation, identified the *Helicobacter pylori* bacterium as the real cause did that field evolve to its present-day effective antibiotic treatment (Marshall and Adams 2008).

This section reviews the evolution of ED treatment approaches and programs in view of the factors just described and offers an appreciation of the expanding concept of EDs and newer approaches to treatment. The convention used herein considers EDs to be syndromes involving psychological and medical components, not simply disordered eating as exemplified by Roman-era gluttony or medieval asceticism through fasting. Although AN is the least common of these disorders, it was historically the first described, with a wide variety of treatment methods employed over the centuries. The term *anorexia nervosa* as it is commonly used in English implies a disorder that generally moves from voluntary onset into involuntary continuation. An understanding of EDs in the twenty-first century is greatly assisted by an appreciation of their history, lest the current diagnostic criteria and treatment methods be considered as arising *de novo* like Aphrodite from the sea, fully formed and enduring.

Anorexia Nervosa

Early Days

A convenient starting point for understanding AN in the modern era is the two cases described by Morton in 1689 (Pearce 2004). Richard Morton was a distinguished seventeenth-century physician who had the perspicacity to differentiate these two cases from the more common wasting disorders of his age, the most common being tuberculosis. He recognized that "nervous consumption" and "cares and passions of the mind" contributed to the patients' emaciation, which was different from most cases of medically caused wasting.

We can trace our modern understanding of AN to almost-simultaneous publication in 1873 of papers by William Gull, physician to Queen Victoria's son, and Charles Lasègue, a French physician and knight of the Legion of Honor. Gull (1873) offered a still-useful description of the physiological changes of AN, recognizing its emotional origin in "a morbid mental state." His pragmatic treatment approach included frequent small feedings, separation of the patient from the family, and "moral" treatment (psychotherapy), quite an improvement from Morton. Lasègue's (1873) descriptions of familial exhaustion from ineffective use of threats and pleas, patients' lack of recognition of the severity of their illness, and the way "the anorexia gradually becomes the sole object of preoccupation and conversation," have an almost contemporary sound. He recommended slow treatment, recognizing that a chronic state of illness was highly probable.

Treatment during the century from the 1870s to the 1970s followed an almost random pattern resulting from radical changes in etiological theories of AN that focused first on the body (the pituitary hormones, 1890s), then on the mind (the psychoanalytic heyday, 1920–1960s), and then on the brain's chemistry (neurotransmitters, 1965–1980). Instead of a systematic and logical gradual increase in understanding AN, treatments followed the most prominent and popular theories of origin of the day.

Neuroendocrinology to the Forefront

No new treatment strategies were advocated until about 1914, when Simmonds published his famous paper on postpartum pituitary necrosis (Birch 1974). The similarities in cachectic appearance between pituitary necrosis and AN led to confidence that the origin of AN had been found. As a result, AN jumped into medical textbooks as being of endocrine origin, where it remained until about 1930 and still continued at times afterward to be considered of medical origin, with treatments that followed *pari passu*. The assumption that AN was of endocrine origin led to its treatment by endocrine replacement, which was not generally available until later decades. Psychological treatments were considered unnecessary. Despite this emphasis on a medical origin, the concept of a wandering uterus being somehow involved kept coming in and out of the etiological picture, resulting in nonmedical but opaque treatments. Only women of childbearing age could develop AN, so males need not apply.

Psychoanalytic Theories and Treatments

In the period from about 1940 to 1965, AN again jumped textbooks, from medical into those of psychodynamic theory and consequent forms of psychodynamic treatment. The case analysis of Ellen West, whom Binswanger considered to have schizophrenia, probably represented a woman with BN (Bray 2001). In 1950, Nemiah described a large series of female patients with AN; he considered their disorder to have arisen in a psychoneurotic setting, perhaps with obsessive-compulsive traits. Parents, especially mothers, were the primary culprits. He found a common feature to be a setting of overprotectiveness leading to dependence and hostility in the developing child, who remained infantile in emotional development. In 1961, Blitzer and colleagues offered a florid description of the context in which AN developed:

> Preconscious and conscious fantasies relating to food and eating included animistic ideas about food, delusions that certain kinds of foods were poisonous, fear of oral impregnation and gastric pregnancies, idea of anal birth,

orally aggressive and sometimes cannibalistic impulses, and the equation of not eating with a lifelong childlike dependent status. (p. 369)

To undo and remediate this nexus required extensive psychodynamic treatment. Psychodynamic theories and psychodynamic psychotherapy treatment methods proliferated and splintered; as a result, many nails protruded from the assumptive theoretical floor, and many carpenters were needed to hammer them back in. Psychodynamic approaches to origin included ego psychology, object relations theory, interpersonal theories, attachment theory, self-psychology, and family systems theory as well as classical psychoanalytic theories. A paucity of evidence for the therapeutic benefit of any of these theories exists.

Pendulum Swings From All Mind to All Brain

The 1963 Nobel Prizes in Physiology or Medicine (recipients Euler, Hodgkin, and Huxley) and 1970 (Katz, Von Euler, and Axelrod) signaled that heady days were ahead to explain many psychiatric disorders as a result of neurotransmitter dysfunction. Theories of the neurochemical origin of AN led to treatment trials of newly described neuroleptics and other medications that promoted eating. These included early antipsychotics—initially chlorpromazine—but later expanded to other first- and second-generation antipsychotics, antihistamines, serotonin reuptake inhibitors, dual-action antidepressants, and marijuana. These treatments were based largely on the belief that if patients would eat more and gain weight, all would be well—or at least better.

This treatment approach led to mixed results. Some patients increased their eating and weight with benefit and partial improvement, whereas others ate more but began to induce vomiting because this pharmacological intrusion provoked their most feared behavior of overeating and becoming fat. Some patients who were unwilling to challenge their overvalued beliefs "ate their way out of the hospital" and relapsed soon after discharge. Currently, theories that abnormal neurotransmitter function, especially in serotonin, predisposes people to developing AN continue to be incompletely understood and unproven. More recent studies have promoted olanzapine and other second-generation antipsychotics/neuroleptics as treatment for AN. Their use as monotherapy is based on the assumption that improved eating and weight gain are the core of treatment.

Integrative and Pragmatic Approaches to Treatment

In the 1960s and 1970s, British clinicians, especially Arthur Crisp and Gerald Russell, and Hilde Bruch in the United States, began approaching the origin of AN more agnostically—or at least, considered theories of its origin to be less rigid. Crisp and Kalucy (1973) believed that adolescents with AN had existential fears of maturation, and Bruch (1973) considered family dysfunction to be common, encouraging increased self-initiative and more accurate identification of bodily states. Clinical case descriptions enlarged the field to include males. Treatments recommended by these authors harkened back to Gull and Lasègue by combining nurse-supervised refeeding with less theoretical psychotherapy, with the goals of persuading patients to change their distorted perception of fatness and challenging patients' fear of becoming fat. Their treatment programs, with good statistical documentation and follow-up studies, offered the first evidence of improved outcome from the natural course of illness.

In the 1980s and onward, intensive hospital-based, integrative, multidisciplinary team approaches to serious cases of AN provided evidence that improvement was possible in most patients and that remission was possible in some. Many studies found long-term outcomes of one-third remitted, one-third stably improved, and one-third chronically and severely ill. All of these programs that demonstrated substantial improvement utilized a team approach (i.e., psychiatrist, psychologist, nutritionist, nurse, social worker, educator); an agreement to use a common psychotherapeutic method (often cognitive-behavioral therapy [CBT]), with extended treatment as needed; and a stepwise progression to less intensive treatment settings (e.g., inpatient, residential care, day program, outpatient follow-up). The program at Johns Hopkins has shown the benefits of rapid refeeding and sequential steps in successful treatment. Unfortunately, reduced funding for fully adequate treatment of AN has resulted in premature discharges leading to increased relapses and readmissions.

CBT appears to be the most effective method of psychotherapy for AN and to contribute substantially to improved outcome, but evidence is less well proven than in BN, largely because hospitalized patients with AN are initially too ill to benefit from a manualized evidence-based psychotherapy, and random assignment to varying psychotherapy methods is difficult with inpatients of varying chronicity and severity. Nonetheless, CBT appears to be the most useful psychotherapy for a programmatic team approach to AN treatment.

Broadening of the Treatment Mission

Five developments have led to a broadening of AN treatment:

1. The treatment of AN, in most cases, involves also treating a cluster of comorbid disorders, both psychiatric and medical. Pure food-restricting AN typically involves treating two or three comorbid psychiatric diag-

noses, most commonly depressive, anxiety, obsessive-compulsive state or trait, substance abuse, and personality disorders (especially those of the Cluster C subtype, with sensitive, persevering, anxious traits).

2. Treatment of a patient involves also treating their family or significant others in varying intensities. Treasure et al. (2010) documented the tremendous burden faced by caregivers of patients with AN and the need for respite care, as well as formal family therapy at times, without any assumptions that families are pathogenic. At a minimum, families require education and support.

3. Innovative approaches have shown that less restrictive home environments, with suitable family training and interaction with clinicians, may be suitable for treatment of even moderately severe AN in teens.

4. At times, the environment, avocation, or vocation of a patient with AN needs to be modified.

5. Medical comorbidities abound in patients with AN. Long-term complications involve a surprising degree of bone mineral density deficiencies (even in males) and persistent gastrointestinal problems. Short-term medical problems may be divided into self-ameliorating (e.g., bradycardia, hypothermia) and urgent/emergent (e.g., electrolyte abnormalities, arrhythmia) signs.

Bulimia Nervosa: A Disorder Hiding in Plain Sight

Few scientific publications have changed the field of psychiatry as quickly or substantially as Gerald Russell's 1979 contribution, "Bulimia Nervosa: An Ominous Variant of Anorexia Nervosa." Clinicians since have shaken their heads, asking why BN had neither been noticed nor described prior to this, which serves to remind us that recognition of new syndromes through keen observation of clinical psychopathology is still possible. On a positive note, despite its relatively recent description and acceptance as a serious ED, treatment for BN came along quickly and convincingly, perhaps for several reasons. Cases of BN are considerably more prevalent than those of AN. They are usually not as severe in terms of medical comorbidity and are less likely to require inpatient treatment; therefore, they are more suitable for rigorous evidence-based studies, especially random assignment to contrasting treatments.

Beck developed CBT in the 1960s, convincingly demonstrating it to be as effective as antidepressants for the treatment of nonpsychotic depressive disorders. Fairburn et al. (1997) were among the first to apply CBT to the treatment of BN; in the 1980s, they demonstrated it to be effective for BN, and by the early to mid-1990s, CBT had become the most convincingly proven psychotherapy for the disorder. To this day, it has rigorous support for the treatment of BN. Analogues of CBT, such as dialectic behavioral therapy and interpersonal psychotherapy, have also been effective, especially in patients with variants of BN, such as borderline personality disorder. These evidence-based therapies often are employed in a group setting, not merely as an economic convenience but also to utilize group support and challenge. The National Institute for Health and Care Excellence in Great Britain requires CBT as the first line of treatment for BN, with other approaches used only if needed for variant disorders. It has given CBT an A rating for the treatment of BN, a designation indicating superiority to other psychological treatments or medications.

For a brief period of time, monotherapy treatment of BN with selective serotonin reuptake inhibitors was in vogue. However, temporary decreases in the frequency of binge eating and purging may revert when the medication is discontinued. Antidepressants may have a role in treating comorbid depressive disorders that accompany BN, but by themselves are inadequate. Monotherapy with psychopharmacological agents primarily reflects a failure to understand the psychopathology of BN. Its entranced morbid fear of fatness leads to dieting, but without the persevering traits of AN that lead to substantial weight loss. The psychopathologies of both AN and BN often include perceptual distortion and overvaluation of the benefits of slimming, as well as a morbid fear of becoming fat.

Although BN treatment should not be oversimplified, and success is not assured in all cases, it has come along much more quickly, and with less psychodynamic baggage, than AN treatment. Patients with BN and comorbid suicidality or severe hypokalemia, or those whose illness is refractory to outpatient treatment, may still need inpatient admission. The subtype of AN with binge-purge features requires a combination of approaches for food-restricting AN and for BN. Binge-purge variants of AN often present with even more comorbid psychological diagnoses than food-restricting AN or BN individually.

Long-term follow-up of BN has revealed variations in the illness trajectory over time. The most common finding is that, prior to their established pattern of BN, about half of patients attempted or actually achieved significant weight loss. AN—either the full disorder or a subclinical form—frequently precedes BN. People with BN appear to lack the persevering traits of food-restricting AN. When their foot is "off the brake" of restrained eating, especially after using alcohol, they engage in binge episodes that short-circuit their attempt at significant weight loss.

Binge-Eating Disorder:
A Late-Comer but a True Eating Disorder

BED has been recognized as a true ED since about the mid-1990s, again, making many wonder how such an obvious disorder had been overlooked.

Its late recognition has been due primarily to assumptions that binge eating without purging, especially in obese individuals, represented hedonic over-eating, lack of willpower, or gluttony. Again, astute clinical inquiry into the presence of psychopathology led to recognition of BED as a true malady. Good phenomenological inquiry is at the heart of syndrome recognition.

Lessons learned from the benefits of CBT in BN were quickly applied to patients with BED, with moderate success. The core of BED treatment includes several facets not dissimilar to BN treatment: interrupting the abnormal binge-eating behavior; challenging the person's ingrained sense of helplessness in the face of relentless binge-eating urges, usually in the service of improving abnormal mood states; and developing new strategies to deal with life's challenges. Although CBT alone may at times be sufficient, BED is the most likely of the three major recognized EDs to require concomitant use of antidepressants. Successful treatment may also require subsequent decision making about remaining obesity, which is sometimes of a morbid degree. Bariatric surgeons generally require patients to prove their BED symptoms have been absent for about 1 year before they will accept them for surgery, a not unreasonable demand. At times, otherwise successful bariatric surgery is undone by postoperative relapse into binge eating. Therefore, good follow-up of patients previously diagnosed with BED or BN is essential after bariatric surgery.

Other Eating Disorders

Other variants of abnormal eating combined with psychopathological states may yet become accepted as EDs. There has always been tension between "lumpers" and "splitters," contrasting those who more broadly group clinical states together as EDs with those who use a more narrow definition to split off each specific clinical presentation. For example, patients with purging disorder, in the experience of many clinicians, have some degree of unwanted driven eating prior to purging; although to an external observer the amount of food consumed may be modest and not typical of BN binges, it is unacceptable to the person. Whether this will turn out to be truly its own ED, split off from that of BN (or of the binge-purge type of AN), or lumped together remains to be seen.

ARFID, the catch-all diagnosis employed by DSM-5 (American Psychiatric Association 2013), presents other problems. Unless the ED category is expanded beyond conventional boundaries to include abnormal eating without an overvalued drive for thinness, morbid fear of fatness, and associated distortion of body image, it lacks syndromic integrity with current understanding of what an ED is. Children younger than about 7 years do not internalize a sociocultural drive for thinness. An ED diagnosis, by convention, requires an abnormal mental state as well as disordered eating, with functional impairment of a reasonable duration. Many children have abnormal eating but do not necessarily have an ED. A separate category of abnormal eating in future diagnostic manuals may be helpful without invoking an ED designation. Time will tell.

Evidence-Based Treatment Parameters

Reversing Nutritional Insufficiencies

Treatment for EDs has predominantly focused on interrupting the abnormal behaviors associated with eating habits (restriction, binge eating, purging), reversing physical and metabolic abnormalities caused by either the malnutrition itself or the behaviors (predominantly electrolyte abnormalities), and attempting to alter the underlying ED psychopathology and treat any psychiatric comorbidities.

In predominantly restricting EDs marked by significant starvation, nutritional rehabilitation most concretely reverses the physical and metabolic effects of malnutrition. Multiple studies have demonstrated resolution of starvation and metabolic derangements via this approach (Keys et al. 1950; Westmoreland et al. 2016). Other arguments for nutritional rehabilitation include data from studies that show low weight on presentation to be associated with a poor outcome (Herzog et al. 2004; Hsu et al. 1979; Sly and Bamford 2011), higher BMI at the start of treatment to be associated with an improved outcome (Hebebrand et al. 1996; Howard et al. 1999; Morgan and Russell 1975; Zipfel et al. 2000), and persistent low weight following treatment to be associated with higher readmission rates and relapse (Baran et al. 1995; Steinhausen et al. 2008). Thus, improving the nutritional status of patients with EDs continues to be a primary, albeit not isolated, focus of treatment.

More recently, recognition that low weight itself is inadequate to identify and evaluate the severity of ED pathology or predict its associated sequelae has complicated this approach. The phenomenon of acute starvation and medical complications in patients who "don't look thin" is well known (Peebles et al. 2010; Whitelaw et al. 2014), yet an obvious bias exists toward people whose body shape changes visibly indicate their nutritional insufficiency. Individuals with an ED who do not appear underweight are identified less quickly, resulting in a longer duration of illness before treatment (Lebow et al. 2015). This bias could narrow the applicability of study results if care is not taken to adequately include these patients. The description of BN as "hiding in plain sight" and the delay in recognizing BED illustrate the delay in recognizing the malnutrition of EDs in people who do not appear outwardly starved by body size. New inclusion in diagnostic manuals of "atypical" AN attempts to recognize the severity of EDs "hidden" behind the appearance of normal weight; however, even the definition of inadequate weight in "typical" AN is somewhat problematic, because consensus on how to calculate a target body weight (Lebow et al. 2018) is lacking. This may result in diagnostic error when assigning patients to either typical or atypical disease (Forman et al. 2014). In addition, many descriptive studies find higher rates of atypical AN than likely justifies nomenclature suggesting scarcity, with studies within specialty treatment centers reporting 25% (Sawyer et al. 2016) to 34% (Forman et al. 2014) and larger epidemiological studies reporting 3–4 times (Stice et al. 2013) and up to 10 times (Hammerle et al. 2016) as many patients meeting criteria for atypical AN.

Resolution of Psychopathology and Comorbid Psychiatric Conditions

Keys et al.'s (1950) original starvation study demonstrated that nutritional rehabilitation can lead to changes in more than just medical sequelae, including improvements in depression, anxiety, irritability, concentration, and social interactions, thus recognizing that improving the body does, in fact, improve the mind. Much of the treatment research in EDs has focused on adults with low-weight AN and has usually shown improvements in ED and comorbid psychiatric pathologies (Channon and de Silva 1985; Meehan et al. 2006; Pollice et al. 1997). The specific linking of weight gain with psychological improvement is sometimes difficult to evaluate because many studies do not directly evaluate this connection. Early results were more mixed, with some showing a direct correlation (Eckert et al. 1982), others showing weight changes not being associated with psychological changes (Coulon et al. 2009; Mattar et al. 2012), and still others showing mixed results (Kawai et al. 2008; Laessle et al. 1988). With regard to severe and enduring AN in adults, Touyz et al. (2013) demonstrated an approach that did not specifically emphasize weight gain as directly but still resulted in improvements in eating and comorbid psychiatric psychopathologies. However, patients did, in general, gain weight, and their nutrition improved.

Family-based treatment for children and adolescents with EDs has shown improvements in both ED and comorbid psychiatric pathology (Le Grange et al. 1992, 2014; Lock et al. 2005), with some data showing that patients with greater eating psychopathology and particularly binge-purge subtypes of AN (considered more severe in pathology) benefited to an even greater degree from nutritional rehabilitation (Accurso et al. 2014; Eisler et al. 2000; Le Grange et al. 1992; Lock et al. 2006). Furthermore, even early weight gain trajectory (a proxy for total nutritional rehabilitation) can predict overall outcome (Accurso et al. 2014). However, some studies still show improvement in eating and comorbid psychiatric psychopathologies without as robust a change in nutrition restoration (Robin et al. 1999). Overall, the data, hough murky at times, suggest that nutritional rehabilitation is an important consideration for treating not only the physical sequelae of EDs but also underlying psychopathology and comorbid psychiatric conditions.

Early Intervention

Viewed through the medical lens of "disease staging," the identification of disease and provision of early intervention are usually linked with improved outcomes. Although consensus on a rubric for staging ED severity has been difficult to achieve, overall data conclude that early treatment is beneficial, with most descriptive studies supporting the conclusion that a longer duration of illness is associated with more severe medical complications, predicts a worse outcome, and is associated with higher relapse rates. Thus, aside from prevention strategies, early intervention is the best way to treat EDs (Berends et al. 2018).

Historically, data have suggested that younger age at onset is associated with more severe ED-related obsessions and comorbid psychiatric conditions. However, some have suggested that the severity of illness in younger patients may, in fact, be the result of delayed identification and a longer duration of illness prior to first treatment (Neubauer et al. 2014). Recent data have supported this finding, showing that the duration of illness itself (and not age) indicates a higher risk of relapse (Berends et al. 2018).

Treasure and Russell (2011) presented a cogent description of the potential theoretical framework behind the idea of early intervention, particularly regarding the developmental process that takes place in the brains of young people. The malnutrition resulting from EDs comes at a time when tremendous developmental changes are occurring in the brain. The loss of brain matter itself interrupts the normal maturation process. The optimal hormonal milieu is also lost, because steroid hormone synthesis depends on adequate substrate, namely cholesterol. Disruption of this milieu impacts areas of the brain involved in self-regulation, impulsivity, mood, and excitability. Finally, animal models have demonstrated the impact of disordered eating on the sensitization of reward pathways within the developing brain, which results in progressive cementing of those pathways over time (Lutter and Nestler 2009; Treasure et al. 2010). This suggests that early intervention may be the only way to truly reverse these paths.

References

Accurso EC, Ciao AC, Fitzsimmons-Craft EE, et al: Is weight gain really a catalyst for broader recovery? The impact of weight gain on psychological symptoms in the treatment of adolescent anorexia nervosa. Behav Res Ther 56:1–6, 2014

American Psychiatric Association: Diagnostic and Statistical Manual of Mental Disorders, 5th Edition. Arlington, VA, American Psychiatric Association, 2013

Anderluh MB, Tchanturia K, Rabe-Hesketh S, Treasure J: Childhood obsessive-compulsive personality traits in adult women with eating disorders: defining a broader eating disorder phenotype. Am J Psychiatry 160(2):242–247, 2003

Baran SA, Weltzin TE, Kaye WH: Low discharge weight and outcome in anorexia nervosa. Am J Psychiatry 152:1070–1072, 1995

Berends T, Boonstra N, van Elburg A: Relapse in anorexia nervosa: a systematic review and meta-analysis. Curr Opin Psychiatry 31(6):445–455, 2018

Birch CA: Simmond's disease. Morris Simmonds 1855–1925. Practitioner 212(1271):737, 1974

Blitzer JR, Rollins SN, Blackwell A: Children who starve themselves: anorexia nervosa. Psychosom Med 23:369–382, 1961

Bray A: The silence surrounding Ellen West: Binswanger and Foucalt. JBSP 32(2):12, 2001

Bruch H: Eating Disorders: Obesity, Anorexia Nervosa and the Person Within. New York, Basic Books, 1973

Channon S, de Silva WP: Psychological correlates of weight gain in patients with anorexia nervosa. J Psychiatr Res 19:267–271, 1985

Crisp AH, Kalucy RS: The effect of leucomy in intractable adolescent weight phobia (primary anorexia nervosa). Postgrad Med J 49:883–893, 1973

Coulon N, Jeammet P, Godart N: Social phobia in anorexia nervosa: evolution during the care. L'Encephale 35:531–537, 2009

Eckert ED, Goldberg SC, Halmi KA, et al: Depression in anorexia nervosa. Psychol Med 12:115–122, 1982

Eisler I, Dare C, Hodes M, et al: Family therapy for adolescent anorexia nervosa: the results of a controlled comparison of two family interventions. J Child Psychol Psychiatry 41:727–736, 2000

Espi Forcen F, Espi Forcen C: The practice of holy fasting in the late Middle Ages: a psychiatric approach. J Nerv Ment Dis 203(8):650–653, 2015

Fairburn CG, Welch SL, Doll HA, et al: Risk factors for bulimia nervosa: a community-based case-control study. Arch Gen Psychiatry 54(6):509–517, 1997

Forman SF, McKenzie N, Hehn R, Monge MC: Predictors of outcome at 1 year in adolescents with DSM-5 restrictive eating disorders: report of the National Eating Disorders Quality Improvement Collaborative. Adolesc Health 55(6):750–756, 2014

Gull WW: Anorexia nervosa (apepsia hysterica, anorexia hysterica). Transactions of the Clinical Society of London, 7:22–28, 1873

Hammerle F, Huss M, Ernst V, Bürger A: Thinking dimensional: prevalence of DSM-5 early adolescent full syndrome, partial and subthreshold eating disorders in a cross-sectional survey in German schools. BMJ Open 6(5), 2016

Hebebrand J, Himmelmann GW, Wewetzer C, et al: Body weight in acute anorexia nervosa and at follow-up assessed with percentiles for the body mass index: implications of a low body weight at referral. Int J Eat Disord 19:347–357, 1996

Herzog T, Zeeck A, Hartmann A, Nickel T: Lower targets for weekly weight gain lead to better results in inpatient treatment of anorexia nervosa: a pilot study. Eur Eat Disord Rev 12:164–168, 2004

Howard WT, Evans KK, Quintero-Howard CV, et al: Predictors of success or failure of transition to day hospital treatment for inpatients with anorexia nervosa. Am J Psychiatry 156:1697–1702, 1999

Hsu LK, Crisp AH, Harding B: Outcome of anorexia nervosa. Lancet 1:61–65, 1979

Kawai K, Yamanaka T, Yamashita S, et al: Somatic and psychological factors related to the body mass index of patients with anorexia nervosa. Eat Weight Disord 13:198–204, 2008

Keys A, Brozek J, Henschel A, et al: The Biology of Human Starvation. Minneapolis, MN, University of Minnesota Press, 1950

Laessle RG, Schweiger U, Pirke KM: Depression as a correlate of starvation in patients with eating disorders. Biol Psychiatry 23:719–725, 1988

Lasègue EC: De l'anorexie hysterique. Arch Gen Med 1:385–403, 1873

Le Grange D, Eisler I, Dare C, Russell G: Evaluation of family treatments in adolescent anorexia nervosa: a pilot study. Int J Eat Disord 12:347–357, 1992

Le Grange D, Accurso EC, Lock J, et al: Early weight gain predicts outcome in two treatments for adolescent anorexia nervosa. Int J Eat Disord 47:124–129, 2014

Lebow J, Sim LA, Kransdorf LN: Prevalence of a history of overweight and obesity in adolescents with restrictive eating disorders. J Adolesc Health 56(1):19–24, 2015

Lebow J, Sim LA, Accurso EC: Is there clinical consensus in defining weight restoration for adolescents with anorexia nervosa? Eat Disord 26(3):270–277, 2018

Lock J, Agras WS, Bryson S, Kraemer HC: A comparison of short- and long-term family therapy for adolescent anorexia nervosa. J Am Acad Child Adolesc Psychiatry 44:632–639, 2005

Lock J, Couturier J, Bryson S, Agras S: Predictors of dropout and remission in family therapy for adolescent anorexia nervosa in a randomized clinical trial. Int J Eat Disord 39:639–647, 2006

Lutter M, Nestler EJ: Homeostatic and hedonic signals interact in the regulation of food intake. J Nutr 139:629–632, 2009

Marshall B, Adams PC: Helicobacter pylori: a Nobel pursuit? Can J Gastroenterol 22(11):895–896, 2008

Mattar L, Thiebaud MR, Huas C, et al: Depression, anxiety and obsessive-compulsive symptoms in relation to nutritional status and outcome in severe anorexia nervosa. Psychiatry Res 200(2–3):513–517, 2012

Meehan KG, Loeb KL, Roberto CA, Attia E: Mood change during weight restoration in patients with anorexia nervosa. Int J Eat Disord 39:587–589, 2006

Miller MN, Pumariega AJ: Culture and eating disorders: a historical and cross-cultural review. Psychiatry 64(2):93–110, 2001

Morgan HG, Russell GF: Value of family background and clinical features as predictors of long term outcome in anorexia nervosa: four-year follow up study of 41 patients. Psychol Med 5:355–371, 1975

Morris PF, Szabo CP: Meanings of thinness and dysfunctional eating in black South African females: a qualitative study. Afr J Psychiatry (Johannesbg) 16(5):338–342, 2013

Nemiah JC: Anorexia nervosa: a clinical study. Medicine (Baltimore) 29(3):225–268, 1950

Neubauer K, Weigel A, Daubmann A, et al: Paths to first treatment and duration of untreated illness in anorexia nervosa: are there differences according to age of onset. Eur Eat Disord Rev 22:292–298, 2014

Pearce JM: Richard Morton: the origins of anorexia nervosa. Eur Neurol 52(4):191–192, 2004

Peebles R, Hardy KK, Wilson JL, Lock JD: Are diagnostic criteria for eating disorders markers of medical severity? Pediatrics 125(5):e1193–e1201, 2010

Pollice C, Kaye WH, Greeno CG, Weltzin TE: Relationship fo depression, anxiety, and obsessionality to state of illness in anorexia nervosa. Int J Eat Disord 21:367–376, 1997

Robin AL, Siegel PT, Moye AW, Gilroy M, et al: A controlled comparison of family versus individual therapy for adolescents with anorexia nervosa. J Am Acad Child Adolesc Psychiatry 38:1482–1489, 1999

Russell G: Bulimia nervosa: an ominous variant of anorexia nervosa. Psychol Med 9:429–448, 1979

Sawyer SM, Whitelaw M, Le Grange D, et al: Physical and psychological morbidity in adolescents with atypical anorexia nervosa. Pediatrics 137(4), 2016

Schaumberg K, Zerwas S, Goodman E, et al: Anxiety disorder symptoms at age 10 predict eating disorder symptoms and diagnoses in adolescence. J Child Psychol Psychiatry 60(6):686–696, 2019

Sly R, Bamford B: Why are we waiting? The relationship between low admission weight and end of treatment weight outcomes. Eur Eat Disord Rev 19:407–410, 2011

Steinhausen HS, Grigoroiu-Serbanescu M, Boyadjieva S, et al: Course and predictors of rehospitalization in adolescent anorexia nervosa in a multisite study. Int J Eat Disord 41:29–36, 2008

Stice E, Marti CN, Rohde P: Prevalence, incidence, impairment, and course of the proposed DSM-5 eating disorder diagnoses in an 8-year prospective community study of young women. J Abnorm Psychol 122(2):445–557, 2013

Touyz S, Le Grange D, Lacey H, et al: Treating severe and enduring anorexia nervosa: a randomized controlled trial. Psychol Med 43:2501–2511, 2013

Treasure J, Russell G: The case for early intervention in anorexia nervosa: theoretical exploration of maintaining factors. Br J Psychiatry 199:5–7, 2011

Treasure J, Claudino AM, Zucker N: Eating disorders. Lancet 375:583–593, 2010

Westmoreland P, Krantz MJ, Mehler PS: Medical complications of anorexia nervosa and bulimia nervosa. Am J Med 129(1):30–37, 2016

Whitelaw M, Gilbertson H, Lee KJ, Sawyer SM: Restrictive eating disorders among adolescent inpatients. Pediatrics 134(3):e758–e764, 2014

Zipfel S, Lowe B, Reas DL, et al: Long-term prognosis in anorexia nervosa: lessons from a 21 year follow-up study. Lancet 355:721–722, 2000

2

Basic Principles of Ethics

Kaila Rudolph, M.D., M.P.H., M.B.E.
Rebecca Weintraub Brendel, M.D., J.D.

THE care of patients with severe eating disorders (EDs) often involves both psychiatric expertise to treat the underlying ED and medical expertise to address any complications, such as electrolyte disturbances and refeeding syndrome. The burden of concurrent medical and psychiatric illness is immense. Differences in perspectives across diverse medical specialties and the interpersonal dynamics between patients, families, and care team members can lead to the development of moral dilemmas. *Moral dilemmas* arise when two or more core ethical principles or considerations are in conflict, and no solution can be found in which all moral obligations are met (Kalvemark et al. 2004). Moral dilemmas are common in the care of patients with EDs and present complex clinical challenges (Matusek and Wright 2010). They commonly center around concerns with coercive treatment practices, ranging from involuntary hospitalization and feeding to the restriction of exercise and surveillance of mealtime and bathroom behaviors (Matusek and Wright 2010). Moral challenges in ED treatment may be addressed via implementation of evidence-based clinical practice recommendations, interdisciplinary collaboration, and analysis of case-by-case factual and moral considerations (Matusek and Wright 2010). Moral dilemmas are an "inherent and inseparable part of good clinical medicine," and medical practitioners should recognize and manage the ethical dilemmas that arise within their practice (Singer et al. 2001).

Clinical ethics is a core component of medicine and is broadly defined as a discipline concerned with the moral dilemmas and choices faced by health care providers in routine clinical practice (Pellegrino 1993). Clinical ethics may include normative ethical considerations, which describe how medical providers ought to act and which treatment recommendations might be morally permissible under specific clinical circumstances (Beauchamp and Childress 2013). Descriptive ethical considerations are also important and may include data and accounts of how providers practice ethics and the actions that are deemed morally permissible by medical professionals (Beauchamp and Childress 2013). The American Medical Association (AMA; 2016) has outlined core principles of clinical ethics to guide physician conduct in clinical encounters. These guidelines emphasize the importance of providing competent, respectful patient care that is informed by patient preferences and accessible across patient populations.

This chapter uses a clinical case to exemplify practical ethical considerations. Given the severity of the medical challenges encountered in individuals with anorexia nervosa (AN), the clinical case focuses on this specific ED. However, the general ethical principles introduced are broadly applicable to the treatment of other EDs (e.g., bulimia nervosa [BN], avoidant/restrictive food intake). Our aim for this chapter is help psychiatrists optimize their ability to identify, systematically approach, and appropriately manage moral dilemmas in ED care with use of available interdisciplinary and ethical consultation resources.

Clinical Vignette: Ms. A.L.

As the consulting psychiatrist working in a community hospital, you receive a call from a general internist colleague who informs you that her service has admitted Ms. A.L., a 21-year-old female with a history of AN, restricting subtype, diagnosed at age 15 years. Her present BMI is 14. She has a history of excessive exercise, and her memberships at several local exercise facilities have been revoked due to concern for her health. She also restricts her caloric intake on a daily basis and reports she ingests <500 calories per day. Ms. A.L. is known to you from a prior medical hospitalization, and she has been treated at the local interdisciplinary outpatient ED clinic. She has also requested discharge prior to completing two prior inpatient ED treatments.

Ms. A.L. was brought to the hospital by her mother, who found her after Ms. A.L. had collapsed in the family living room. On admission to the general internal medicine service, Ms. A.L. was noted to be hypoglycemic, bradycardic, and hypotensive. Intravenous fluid resuscitation and intravenous dextrose resolved her hypotension and hypoglycemia. She has pancytopenia, and an echocardiogram demonstrated end-organ damage with an abnormally low left ventricular ejection fraction. Although she requested to leave the hospital, her mother refused to allow her to return home until she received further treatment. Hence, Ms. A.L. agreed to stay at this time. The nutrition and endocrinology teams assessed her and offered her meals consistent with her stated food preferences. She subsequently refused all meals in the hospital. Without nutrition, she is now at risk for recurrent hypotension and hypoglycemia, with worsening end-organ damage, seizure, and death. The team asks you to evaluate Ms. A.L.'s capacity to refuse nutrition.

Foundational Principles in Clinical Ethics

The practice of clinical ethics employs theories and tools to help clinician-ethicists engage in moral reasoning and arrive at moral judgments to address moral dilemmas. Although this chapter focuses on moral theories and reasoning, these are not the only tools in ethical decision making (Haidt 2001). *Moral intuition*, the emergence of sudden moral judgments that bypass moral reasoning and generally carry an affective valence, also plays a role in formulating moral judgments, which are important to consider and acknowledge in the work of clinical ethics (Haidt 2001). Additionally, nonmoral factors, such as financial constraints, resource limitations, and patient engagement with care, are often critical factors for arriving at practical and morally permissible responses to ethical challenges. This chapter focuses on principlism, virtue ethics, and narrative ethics as three core approaches to moral dilemmas.

The moral theories of utilitarianism and deontology are grounded in the value of an action's consequences and the importance of being rational and not treating people as a means to an end, respectively (Beauchamp and Childress 2013). The application of such theories can yield clear moral judgments, but when applied in isolation, they may neglect important moral obligations in clinical ethics (Beauchamp and Childress 2013). Beauchamp and Childress's (2013) principlism theory rests upon four key moral principles to guide ethical decision making: autonomy, beneficence, nonmaleficence, and justice:

1. *Autonomy* refers to one's right to self-governance. It allows capable decision makers to formulate decisions that are consistent with their personal values and preferences. The duty to respect autonomy rests on the assumption that patients are able to formulate capable medical decisions concordant with their values and beliefs.
2. *Beneficence* refers to the promotion of the welfare of others.
3. *Nonmaleficence* refers to the duty not to harm.

4. *Justice* has broad potential applications in clinical ethics and may refer to fairly allocating scarce medical resources and to ensuring that high-quality medical care is accessible across diverse patient populations.

Whereas moral theories require strict adherence to the governing rule undergirding them, pluralist approaches, such as principlism, are based on *prima facie* or self-evident competing considerations that must be specified and balanced to determine morally permissible actions in particular circumstances. To employ a principlist approach in a given clinical case, one must first identify the core moral principles most relevant to the scenario and then consider any conflicting moral obligations. In the case of Ms. A.L., the principles of autonomy, beneficence, and nonmaleficence are both central and in conflict. The team cannot provide the recommended clinical treatment (beneficence) while simultaneously honoring Ms. A.L.'s stated preferences (autonomy). Managing the duty to nonmaleficence is challenging in ED care because the severe health risks of not providing treatment must be weighed against the potential harm of providing involuntary treatment, which may be traumatic for the patient and adversely impact the therapeutic alliance and engagement in care. Conflicting moral duties can be difficult to resolve. One must consider what moral principles may be permissible to override and whether any moral obligations take precedence in a particular clinical scenario (Beauchamp and Childress 2013). Moral judgments made in individual medical ethics cases must be consistent with broader professional obligations, such as those outlined by the AMA, the institution providing medical care, and society as a whole (Beauchamp and Childress 2013).

A common critique of employing a purely principle-based approach to an ethical dilemma is that no objective mechanism exists to prioritize conflicting principles (Matusek and Wright 2010). As a result, medical professionals may prioritize principles that favor their preferred outcome to yield an ethical analysis that supports their personal preference (Matusek and Wright 2010). Given the subjective nature of prioritizing individual ethical principles, professionals must explicitly identify and disclose their personal values relevant to the clinical case and openly document and discuss the decision-making process informing their ethical analysis, while also remembering that the unique preferences of the competent patient must prevail when not overridden by other considerations (Matusek and Wright 2010).

In addition to considering what moral norms ought to be satisfied in the practice of clinical ethics, some moral theories, namely virtue ethics, are concerned with the character traits of health care practitioners acting as moral agents within the medical setting (Gardiner 2003). *Virtues* have been defined as enduring character traits, demonstrated through consistent actions, that enhance the well-being of virtuous agents and the people around them (Gardiner 2003). They have been conceptualized along a continuum, with virtuous traits lying at the mean between two extreme vices (Gardiner 2003). For example, the virtue of compassion would rest between the extremes of callousness and indulgence (Gardiner 2003). Virtues identified as most relevant to the practice of medicine include compassion, trustworthiness, integrity, discernment, and conscientiousness (Beauchamp and Childress 2013; Gardiner 2003). An additional virtue that has been recognized is *tolerance*, which is the valuing of unique viewpoints, cultures, and personal preferences that inform how people define a life worth living (Matusek and Wright 2010). A virtue ethics approach considers how a practitioner *ought* to be; how a medical professional might act in a situation is determined by the standard of how a virtuous provider would act (Gardiner 2003). Virtue ethics is not a rule-bound approach but, rather, considers standards of virtuous behavior and what sort of person one ought to be, along with internal attitudes, feelings, and reason, with its end result to foster human flourishing (Gardiner 2003).

Virtue ethics has facilitated development of an ethics of care approach, which prioritizes the importance of taking care of others and the centrality of trust and relationships within clinical ethics (Timmons 2013). Relational and compassion-focused ethical approaches move beyond considerations of logic, and what one *should* do, to conceptualize actions based on a range of virtues that may further clarify the moral behaviors embodied by medical professionals (Timmons 2013). Such models allow for the incorporation of provider self-awareness in ethical decision making and highlight the importance of relational influences, including and integrating multiple stakeholder perspectives (Matusek and Wright 2010). A relational emphasis works closely with patients to strengthen the therapeutic alliance and facilitate simultaneous promotion of patient preferences, safety, and well-being (Matusek and Wright 2010). Proactive treatment planning, honest presentation of the rationale for a recommended medical treatment, open discussion of patient resistance to treatment, and provider willingness to negotiate some aspects of care may promote shared decision making (Matusek and Wright 2010). Such behaviors can support affiliative patient–provider relations and reduce the emergence of adversarial interpersonal dynamics between the treatment team and the patient and family (Matusek and Wright 2010).

Patient stories or narratives are an additional tool that has become increasingly implemented in clinical ethics (Montello 2014). *Narrative ethics* is an approach concerned with understanding the stories of patients and families to gain a greater appreciation of how they have arrived at their present ethical dilemma, how they have resolved past moral challenges, and their values and goals (Montello 2014). There are four primary elements in narrative ethics: voice, character, plot, and resolution (Montello 2014). When considering *voice*, ethicists should contemplate the perspective from which the story is told and why the teller has chosen to share this story at this time (Montello 2014). *Character* implores us to consider who is at the center of the story, whose story it is, and the narrative differences between the patient and family members (Montello 2014). *Plot* is concerned with understanding the content of the narrative and identifying areas of acute distress, loss, or disappointment in which patients and families may need help accepting and incorporating difficult events (Montello 2014). *Resolution* refers to helping the patient and family use values, preferences, and past coping strategies to move forward in the struggle they currently face (Montello 2014). The care team supports the patient and family in identifying the morally permissible choices they must consider to determine the least distressing outcome (Montello 2014). Narrative approaches can foster empathic understanding of patients and families to strengthen the therapeutic alliance and help formulate patient-centered moral judgments (Montello 2014).

Engaging a pluralism of theory and method in clinical ethics empowers clinician-ethicists by creating a number of possible ethical courses of action from which the patient can choose according to his or her unique characteristics and personal values to the best extent possible in any given clinical situation. A moral pluralism approach to clinical ethics, in which clinician-ethicists are not bound to one moral theory but rather may use a diverse range of moral principles and tools, may further avoid the risk of "cherry picking" the approach that most serves the outcome desired by the clinical ethics team. This ensures that a multitude of approaches is engaged in every case. We recognize that some ethicists prefer and adhere to approaches based on one moral theory; however, we maintain that broad foundational ethical knowledge can facilitate employment of a flexible and diverse range of ethical skills tailored to clinical cases. This approach may enhance interdisciplinary team collaborations and assist with the practical implementation of these ethical frameworks and tools in diverse contexts, such as the care of patients with medical and psychiatric challenges.

Concurrent Medical and Psychiatric Challenges

Patients with medical and psychiatric illnesses experience unique ethical challenges. A recent survey of consultation-liaison psychiatrists revealed that 67.4% found that ethical issues had a moderate to profound impact on their clinical work (Bourgeois 2006). The most commonly encountered ethical dilemmas involved challenges with decisional capacity and informed consent, with additional challenges including withdrawal of life-sustaining care and psychiatric commitment of medically ill patients (Bourgeois 2006). Moral dilemmas surrounding consent and capacity are central to the practice of psychiatry in the medical setting, and we consider foundational principles to address decisional capacity dilemmas in the following discussion.

Patient-centered care has become a cornerstone of medical practice and is widely recognized as a component of high-quality health care (Barry and Edgman-Levitan 2012). The Institute of Medicine defines *patient-centered care* as being respectful of and responsive to patient needs and allowing the patient's values and goals to guide all health care decisions (Barry and Edgman-Levitan 2012). Respecting patient autonomy is central to this model because it permits decision making that is consistent with a patient's preferences, without interference from external influences, and recognizes that medical treatment determinations depend upon personal value preferences that are outside the medical expertise domain (Beauchamp and Childress 2013). Providing health care that is consistent with patients' goals and values, which is achieved by honoring their treatment decisions, may promote enhanced quality of life and well-being (Pellegrino and Thomasma 1987). Clinicians strive to respect patient autonomy and provide care that is consistent with patients' values and conceptions of a life worth living.

This focus on respect for autonomy represents a shift away from paternalism in medical practice (Matusek and Wright 2010). *Paternalism* is defined as the restriction of one's ability to participate in choices and actions influencing one's care that would serve to promote one's own welfare (Giordano 2007). It generally occurs when medical providers believe they have a better understanding of patients' best interests than the patients do themselves (Kontos 2013). Paternalism often focuses only on the medical benefits and not on the broader concepts of patient benefit, including social, religious, and psychological well-being, encompassed in the ethical principle of beneficence (Kontos 2013). A paternalist approach may lead to involuntary medical treatment in the form of physical and chemical restraints and forced nutrition for psychiatric patients within the medical setting. Because paternalism may not truly reflect beneficent action and may encroach on the responsibility of nonmaleficence, it is not a core ethical principle or justification for involuntary treatment and must be distinguished from beneficence in clinical practice (Kontos 2013). Paternalism may be necessary to restrict the actions of an incapacitated person, but it is misplaced if it limits the freedom of an autonomous agent (Giordano 2007). The distinction between times when paternalism infringes on the rights of an autonomous person and times when it may be necessary for the care of an incapacitated patient reminds us that the duty to respect autonomy rests on the assumption that patients have the capacity to formulate medical decisions concordant with their values and beliefs (Beauchamp and Childress 2013).

To show they have the capacity to make autonomous decisions, patients must demonstrate the ability to give informed consent for a specific medical treatment (Sher and Sermsak 2014). Informed consent requires that the treating professional make a full disclosure of relevant medical information and that the patient demonstrate decisional capacity to make a voluntary, informed choice free from coercion (Sher and Sermsak 2014). Decisional capacity comprises four components: the patient's ability to 1) clearly state a preferred treatment option, 2) understand relevant medical information, 3) appreciate how this medical information relates to a specific medical condition and its treatment course, and 4) provide a rationale for choosing the preferred medical treatment (Appelbaum 2007).

Patients who have decisional capacity and the ability to give informed consent may refuse medical treatment, including emergency medical treatment (Glezer and Brendel 2010). In contrast, those who lack decisional capacity and cannot provide informed consent require the help of a surrogate decision maker or health care proxy (Torke et al. 2008). Initiation of involuntary treatment for incapable patients is common in clinical practice and raises important ethical challenges, given the need to balance duties to beneficence (the health benefits of treatment) with nonmaleficence (the harm of forced medical interventions) (Giordano 2007; Kendall 2014). The involuntary treatment of incapable patients is generally a last-resort option reserved for cases of significant risk to survival in the absence of less intrusive treatment alternatives (Elzakkers et al. 2018). Ethical justifications for involuntary treatment generally argue that the benefits of the proposed medical intervention are significant, provide lifesaving care and enhancement to future quality of life, and outweigh the potential harm of providing involuntary care that is inconsistent with the person's stated preferences (Giordano 2007). Conversely, it may be argued that coercive treatment violates our ethical obligation to provide dignified, compassionate patient care and that the need to respect patient preferences and nonmaleficence outweighs our obligation to beneficence (Giordano 2007). Involuntary treatment has been associated with patients' experiences of loss of liberty and integrity, and a balance must be found between respectful, compassionate care that acknowledges patient preferences and beneficent care (Johansson and Lundman 2002).

Conflicts between core ethical principles, such as tension between patient autonomy and the physician's obligation to promote beneficence, may produce moral distress in patients, families, and medical teams. *Moral distress* has been defined as the emotional experience that results from being unable to pursue a desired course of clinical action within the setting of institutional constraints (Traudt 2016). Moral distress has been linked to providing care that is deemed harmful to, has no clear medical indication for, and dehumanizes the patient receiving care (Traudt 2016). Self-awareness of the experience of moral distress, the ability to advocate for patient welfare, and a working environment that supports collegial relationships and conflict management help reduce moral distress (Traudt 2016). Psychiatric training provides a skill set that helps practitioners develop a sense of moral agency and a moral community that supports discussions of moral distress and offers potential ethical solutions to emergent moral dilemmas (Traudt 2016). Recognizing and assisting in the management of moral distress is a key role of both psychiatrists and ethicists caring for patients with medical and psychiatric illness.

Requests for capacity evaluations often emerge in the setting of moral dilemmas and distress (Kontos 2013). These evaluations function both to promote enhanced quality of life for autonomous patients who are capable of making medical decisions and to protect patients who lack capacity from the potential harm of making decisions while they are unable to formulate choices consistent with their personal values (Appelbaum 2007).

Returning to the case of Ms. A.L., her medical team members face competing obligations. On the one hand, they have a duty to promote her well-being and health, and to satisfy this, they think providing nutrition is the most appropriate care measure. Conversely, they also have an obligation to respect her values and capable preferences and to consider the impact of treatment on her during both her present admission and her ongoing medical and psychiatric care.

> During your evaluation of Ms. A.L., she is cooperative and engaged with assessment. She is able to demonstrate a detailed understanding of AN, her treatment history, and the reason for her medical admission. She denies that the reason for her fainting was malnutrition, noting that low blood pressure is common in healthy young women her age. She indicates that she has been engaged in her current eating behaviors for many years and does not believe she is at imminent risk of harm should she leave the hospital without further treatment. She is aware of her blood work and echocardiogram findings but minimizes their significance, noting that these are chronic challenges that do not warrant inpatient medical care or significant medical treatment. She reports eating sufficient amounts of food prior to and during her hospitalization. Although she can list the risks and potential benefits of nasogastric feeding, she remarks that this is an inappropriate treatment for her because she believes she has consumed sufficient calories while in the hospital. She indicates she is at low risk of adverse medical outcomes should she continue her current oral consumption without intervention. Although she meets the understanding criterion of the capacity evaluation, you opine that she is incapable of refusing nasogastric tube insertion due to her failure to appreciate the nature of her illness and its impact on her present health and medical

treatment. Her mother is designated as her health care proxy to assist with this decision.

Decisional Capacity in Severe Eating Disorders

The case of Ms. A.L. highlights the complexities present in capacity evaluations of patients with severe EDs. These patients often present as intelligent, articulate people capable of making medical decisions about other conditions and well informed about the medical and psychiatric manifestations of their ED and available treatments (Giordano 2007; Kendall 2014). Consequently, like Ms. A.L., they meet the "understanding" criterion for capacity. Careful evaluation is needed to assess the "appreciation" criterion, however, because this may be influenced by symptoms of the patient's ED, including disordered cognitions about food and body image, more pervasive cognitive impairment related to severe and prolonged malnutrition, and impaired insight into the nature of this life-threatening condition (Elzakkers et al. 2018). At the bedside, appreciation may be evaluated through questions such as, "What are the present concerns with your health?" or "Do you believe you require treatment?" and "What are the potential risks to you if you accept or decline medical treatment?" (Appelbaum 2007). A study investigating decisional capacity in women with AN found that physicians overestimated incapacity in patients with disordered eating (Elzakkers et al. 2018). Psychiatrists should consider using standardized capacity assessment tools to aid in completion of these complex evaluations (Elzakkers et al. 2018). Because EDs can influence patients' sense of self and personal values, obtaining collateral history regarding the patients' preferences during periods of health and acute illness may help assess whether their preferences during severe illness are in keeping with prior capable wishes (Kendall 2014).

Although patients' cognition and underlying ED may affect their capacity, one should not assume they are incapable of consenting to treatment in the absence of a formal capacity evaluation (Giordano 2007). Patients with psychiatric disorders may be capable of making many treatment decisions, and a thorough capacity assessment is required to determine patients' decisional capacity across the continuum of specific medical decisions needed during the course of treatment (Giordano 2007; Kendall 2014). The cognitive impact of malnutrition and the unique phases of illness in the care of persons with EDs may cause changes in their decisional capacity at different stages during the illness (Lauer 1999).

Existing evidence demonstrates cognitive impairments in domains such as working memory, problem solving, and attention in acutely symptomatic patients with AN and BN (Lauer 1999). These cognitive deficits may improve significantly in both conditions when the patient achieves clinical remission (Lauer 1999). Acute impairments in cognitive functioning that may improve with treatment present ethically relevant information supporting dynamic capacity capabilities and the need for serial capacity reevaluations over the course of treatment. Existing evidence also supports the notion that the treatment preferences of patients with EDs may change over time (Guara 2007; Túry et al. 2019).

Capacity assessments do not dispel ethical dilemmas by absolving medical providers of the need to respect patient autonomy and allowing them to proceed with paternalistic treatment initiatives (Kontos 2013). Capacity evaluations are often an initial step in addressing an ethical dilemma. When patients lack decisional capacity for a specific decision, key ethical determinations include appointing a proxy decision maker and identifying morally permissible courses of action, which are discussed in collaboration with the patient, the surrogate decision maker, and the medical team. From an ethical standpoint, it is critical to consider the most appropriate decisional standard to implement for incapable patients with EDs. For incapable persons who have had periods of capacity, psychiatric advance directives and substituted judgment are the preferred decisional standards, given their ability to respect the prior autonomous wishes of the incapacitated patient (Torke et al. 2008). Team members have an ethical obligation to support family members in making decisions consistent with substituted-judgment standards rather than propose medical decisions based upon next-of-kin preferences. Psychiatric advance directives provide written guidance for care preferences in the setting of incapacity, are becoming increasingly used in clinical practice, and are recognized as legal documents in more than 20 states (Swanson 2006). Given the low rates of advance-directive completion, the next of kin may be requested to provide substituted-judgment preferences, which requires health care proxies to formulate medical decisions consistent with the choice the incapacitated person would have made if he or she had the capacity to make the decision (Torke et al. 2008). The most appropriate decisional standard for children, adolescents, and adults with no prior period of capacity or known prior capable-care preferences has been a subject of debate (American Academy of Pediatrics 2016; Torke et al. 2008); although the best-interest standard is widely discussed, uncertainty remains about its most appropriate definition and use in practice (Torke et al. 2008). Some authors have proposed a best-interest standard based on balancing the risks and benefits that a reasonable person would be expected to consider and the use of community standards of people with similar characteristics (Torke et al. 2008).

In the case of Ms. A.L., a determination of incapacity to refuse nutrition is not synonymous with ethical permissibility to proceed with involuntary feeding. Rather, it is the beginning of an ethical deliberation of the potential morally permissible courses of action and should involve Ms. A.L., her family, and the clinical team. Involuntary treatment in ED care is controversial and hinges on patient severity of illness, insight, the degree of compulsory care required, and the risks and benefits of the proposed treatment (Túry et al. 2019). Three common ethical positions on involuntary feeding in ED care include 1) involuntary feeding is ethically permissible as a life-sustaining therapy, 2) involuntary feeding may be harmful but justifiable as a means to facilitate meaningful future treatment engagement, and 3) coercive treatment is ethically impermissible (Giordano 2007).

For those who argue that involuntary feeding is ethically permissible, the need to provide beneficent, life-sustaining medical treatment outweighs any moral duty to nonmaleficence arising from harms inflicted by coercive measures and violating the preferences of the incapacitated person (Kendall 2014; Túry et al. 2019). The high rates of mortality in AN and the clinical duty to protect patients from imminent harm of possible death and starvation are rationales that support compulsory treatment (Kendall 2014; Túry et al. 2019). In such cases, the current requirement for life-sustaining care may be argued to take precedence over the expected adverse impact of involuntary treatment on patient quality of life during and afterward. Others focus on the permissibility of short-term involuntary treatment as a mechanism to restore the person's cognitive functioning and decisional capacity and facilitate reengagement in ED care (Giordano 2007; Túry et al. 2019). Malnourished patients with an ED may be cognitively impaired and unable to meaningfully participate in psychotherapeutic treatment; thus, involuntary feeding may be ethically justified as a short-term intervention to address the malnutrition, with the goal of facilitating the return of decisional capacity and the patient's ability to participate in care (Giordano 2007). Notably, individual treatment experiences are important to take into account (Kendall 2014). Patients with chronic AN who have demonstrated limited personal response to past involuntary ED care may have a risk-benefit analysis skewed toward minimization of suffering given their history of limited treatment benefit (Kendall 2014). Those with concurrent EDs and severe trauma histories or PTSD may experience more severe harm from coercive treatment than do patients with ED and no trauma history, and this must be considered in the treatment risk-benefit analysis (Giordano 2007).

Alternatively, some consider involuntary feeding morally impermissible and fear that the disempowerment and violation of involuntary treatment will intensify the need for control and jeopardize treatment engagement (Giordano 2007). This raises concern that involuntary treatment will intensify ED behaviors by reducing the agency of patients who are already immersed in an illness that exerts control over their environment (Giordano 2007). Consequently, there is concern that involuntary treatment may lead to exacerbation of ED behaviors and the need for recurrent hospitalizations. It may also cause patients to mistrust the treatment team and make them less willing to engage with subsequent clinical care (Giordano 2007).

The literature has debated the clinical outcomes from involuntary ED treatment (Kendall 2014; Túry et al. 2019). Some research highlights the short-term efficacy of compulsory refeeding in AN, noting uncertain long-term efficacy, whereas other research has found benefits from both short- and long-term compulsory treatment with no adverse effect on therapeutic alliance (Kendall 2014; Túry et al. 2019). Given this debate, it remains important to consider how absence of patient insight, limited treatment engagement, and coercive measures may impact ED care. Patient experiences of disempowerment may contribute to care disengagement, limited clinical improvement, and high rates of relapse and disease chronicity, phenomena commonly encountered in ED care (Medeiros 2014). Providers may experience feelings of helplessness, hopelessness, and anxiety, and in an effort to improve care outcomes, may increasingly resort to involuntary treatments (Medeiros 2014). Involuntary feeding efforts generally produce favorable medical results in the short term, which may positively reinforce this strategy (Medeiros 2014), but over time, the desire to maintain control, by both the patient and physician, may contribute to a strained therapeutic alliance and reduce future patient motivation to engage in clinical care, thus potentially impacting long-term treatment outcomes (Medeiros 2014). We must continue to empower patients by incorporating their preferences and values into care even in the setting of decisional incapacity (Giordano 2007). A shift away from outcome-focused ethical frameworks toward virtue and narrative patient-centered approaches may enable recognition of provider countertransference and interpersonal tensions and provide an opportunity to preserve patient empowerment and therapeutic alliance.

For Ms. A.L., an ethics consultation and interdisciplinary team meeting were held to consider the appropriateness of involuntary feeding. The ethics consultants and care team concluded that short-term involuntary feeding was morally permissible for Ms. A.L. at this time. Key factors for this decision included 1) her limited treatment history and the opportunity to offer early intervention care to reduce the likelihood of a chronic illness course; 2) her current inability to engage with treatment in the setting of hypotension, hypoglycemia, and cognitive impairment rendering her incapacitated; and 3) the evidence of end-organ damage thought to present life-threatening risk if refeeding were not initiated in the acute medical setting. The treatment team discussed nasogastric feeding in depth with Ms. A.L. and her mother and promoted the patient's preferences by suggesting use of the smallest-gauge tube to minimize her pain and discomfort, involvement of her outpatient therapist to hold counseling sessions in the hospital, daily meetings with the hospital nutritionist and meals composed of her preferred foods, and provision of recreational activities such as reading and music. Ms. A.L. was aware that sufficient oral intake would facilitate nasogastric tube removal. After 5 days of nasogastric feeding, her caloric intake was sufficient to facilitate transition to oral intake, and she sustained adequate caloric intake during the remainder of her hospitalization. She was discharged to the care of her community ED treatment team.

Obligations to Community and Licensing Boards

As the case of Ms. A.L. shows, patients with EDs require access to diverse treatment modalities to serve their evolving care needs. ED treatment occurs across medical, psychiatric, inpatient, outpatient, and community care settings and spans stages of illness, encompassing goals from prevention to remission and palliation. The chronic relapsing-remitting course of EDs leads to dynamic care needs, with frequent care transitions requiring investment in care coordination. Ethical obligations to promote beneficence and nonmaleficence support the requirement for community and licensing boards to provide accessible, evidence-based treatment across the spectrum of ED care to the range of patient populations affected.

EDs are important considerations for community and licensing boards, because they pose significant public health concerns as evident in both developed and developing countries (Austin 2016). Despite the prevalence of EDs and their associated morbidity and mortality, limited access and engagement in treatment remain a concern across the United States (Hudson et al. 2007). Existing evidence has found that fewer than half of patients with EDs receive treatment during their lifetime (Hudson et al. 2007). This shortage has reverberations for justice from a gender perspective, given that EDs requiring hospitalization are far more common among females than males. Additionally, despite evidence suggesting similar disease prevalence rates across racial groups, racial minority patient populations have significantly reduced lifetime engagement with mental health services, leading to health disparities in ED care (Marques et al. 2011).

To fulfill their ethical obligations to beneficence, nonmaleficence, and justice, licensing boards have an ethical imperative to advocate for equitable models of ED care provision. Increased accessibility may be achieved by offering ED care across multiple levels of health care delivery, including community, hospital, and in-home services, and ensuring that adequate care is covered by a diverse range of insurance policies, including Medicaid, with opportunities to access free care programs and financial aid. Provider education initiatives that promote awareness of available community and academic center ED resources and community and licensing board protocols that allocate care services across lower-resource communities may further support increased care accessibility. Given evidence of racial disparities in care access, community and licensing boards must consider at-risk populations and develop strategic plans to enhance opportunities for engagement and participation in care. The shortage of mental health care providers is a significant barrier to accessible care, and continued expansion of initiatives to fund and train behavioral health specialists with ED expertise is needed. Increasing program accessibility may reduce morbidity and mortality by providing ED care and promoting treatment engagement.

In addition to advocating for equitable care access, community and licensing boards have an ethical imperative to provide patient-centered care that encompasses diverse evidence-based treatments. A broad range of approaches can avoid harms from ineffective treatment and inappropriate resource allocation and subsequent risk of illness progression and involuntary care. Access to multimodal evidence-based treatments that can be tailored to patient care needs may achieve enhanced patient engagement in accordance with respect for persons and the principle of autonomy. In contrast to community care, acute inpatient treatment provides a contained setting where patients with severe illness can receive both voluntary and involuntary care. The transition from acute, involuntary inpatient treatment to nonacute, voluntary community care poses challenges to engagement. Voluntary community programs may encourage engagement by providing care that is adaptable to patient symptomatology through the use of care models centered on patient needs and preferences, including psychotherapy services that utilize motivational interviewing strategies (Matusek and Wright 2010). Care adherence may be promoted by smooth care transitions in which outpatient providers meet with patients prior to hospital discharge.

Community and licensing boards' obligations to beneficence promote extension of care to the implementation of ED prevention programs (Harvard T. H. Chan School of Public Health 2019). Advocacy organizations such as The Harvard Chan School of Public Health's Strategic Training Initiative for the Prevention of Eating Disorders (STRIPED) demonstrate the need for widespread public health efforts to implement ED prevention programming for young adults to reduce the prevalence and adverse health consequences of these disorders for future generations. At the other end of the illness spectrum, persons with treatment-refractory EDs who wish to pursue comfort care measures should have the option of appropriate palliative care services for symptom management and end-of-life care.

Within the current health care infrastructure, pervasive constraints limit the capacity of clinicians and licensing boards to provide care that is consistent with the standards outlined by ethical obligations. Moral obligations to beneficence, nonmaleficence, and justice can also be applied to ED resource allocation strategies. Resource rationing dilemmas occur across different levels of health care. At the community level, allocation dilemmas may pertain to competing moral obligations to invest resources in various populations of patients—healthy, at-risk patients who require prevention programming, patients with new-onset ED who require early intervention care, and those with severe, treatment-refractory illness who require residential programming and palliative care services. Community and licensing board consideration of these moral obligations, with careful weighing of the risks and benefits to patients and communities, is critical for ethical ED resource allocation and treatment. Such moral dilemmas are challenging to identify and address and may benefit from interdisciplinary team and ethics consultation collaboration with medical licensure authorities.

> Ms. A.L. continued to demonstrate chronic symptoms of AN, for which she required intermittent hospitalization with multiple episodes of acute involuntary feeding, completion of three inpatient ED programs, and engagement with outpatient ED care. Nineteen years later, at the age of 40, she again presents to your acute care hospital with weakness and recurrent hypotension and hypoglycemia. She describes her quality of life as very poor in the setting of her ongoing ED and medical challenges. She has informed her physicians that she has already engaged in numerous ED programs and does not wish to undergo further involuntary feeding or aggressive medical interventions because these strategies caused her pain and emotional distress and did not change her overall illness trajectory. Although she does not wish to die, she highlights her quality-of-life limitations, which include fatigue, limited independence, and pain from history of compression fractures. She requests medical care that will allow her to be comfortable and improve her quality of life. She specifically requests a palliative care consult. Collateral history from her outpatient ED team indicates that she has consistently expressed these wishes in the setting of her persistent challenges with poor quality of life.
>
> You and a second psychiatrist both find Ms. A.L. to possess decisional capacity. The ethics committee and interdisciplinary care team meet with her to discuss her treatment course. This time, the ethics consultants and care team conclude it is not morally permissible to initiate involuntary feeding. Key factors in this decision include 1) her history of repeated involuntary feeding interventions and PTSD from involuntary nasogastric feeding, with limited impact on her illness trajectory; 2) her engagement in intensive outpatient and inpatient care interventions with limited impact on her ill-

ness trajectory; and 3) her symptom burden and persistent concerns with low quality of life despite her engagement with outpatient care and prior palliative care consultation. In ethical terms, at this time, the weight of the principle of beneficence in involuntary treatment appears reduced in balance with those of autonomy and nonmaleficence. Her ethical team used person-centered ethical approaches that appealed to the need for compassionate care, prioritization of her prior and current experiences of care, and her goals of minimized suffering and maximized quality of life to arrive at this decision as an ethically permissible treatment option.

Conclusion

This chapter explored foundational principles of medical ethics and aimed to apply them to the complex moral dilemmas encountered in the care of patients with EDs. Psychiatrists providing care to this population have a critical role in resolving moral dilemmas, because their training supports recognition of such dilemmas and distress and management of challenging interpersonal dynamics among teams, patients, and families via effective communication and conflict resolution. The use of person-centered moral tools, such as virtue and narrative ethical principles, complements the skill set of psychiatrists and can promote positive patient–provider interactions, allowing patients to retain a sense of dignity and control in their care. Moral principles can be used to balance the need for equitable, accessible ED care with the reality of the resource allocation challenges faced by providers within the present medical system.

References

American Academy of Pediatrics: Policy statement: Informed consent in decision-making in pediatric practice. Pediatrics 138(2):e20161484, 2016

American Medical Association: AMA Code of Ethics. Chicago, IL, 2016. Available at: https://www.ama-assn.org/about/publications-newsletters/ama-principles-medical-ethics. Accessed July 15, 2020.

Appelbaum P: Assessment of patients' competence to consent to treatment. N Engl J Med 357:1834–1840, 2007

Austin SB: Accelerating progress in eating disorders prevention: a call for policy translation research and training. Eat Disord 24(1):6–19, 2016

Barry MJ, Edgman-Levitan S: Shared decision making: pinnacle of patient-centered care. N Engl J Med 366(9):780–781, 2012

Beauchamp TL, Childress JF: Principles of Biomedical Ethics, 7th Edition. New York, Oxford University Press, 2013

Bourgeois JA: The role of psychosomatic-medicine psychiatrists in bioethics: a survey study of members of the Academy of Psychosomatic Medicine. Psychosomatics 47:520–526, 2006

Elzakkers IFFM, Danner UN, Grisso T, et al: Assessment of mental capacity to consent to treatment in anorexia nervosa: a comparison of clinical judgment and MacCAT-T and consequences for clinical practice. Int J Law Psychiatry 58:27–35, 2018

Gardiner P: A virtue ethics approach to moral dilemmas in medicine. J Med Ethics 29:297–302, 2003

Giordano S: Understanding Eating Disorders: Conceptual and Ethical Issues in the Treatment of Anorexia and Bulimia Nervosa. New York, Oxford University Press, 2007

Glezer A, Brendel RW: Beyond emergencies: the use of physical restraints in medical and psychiatric settings. Harv Rev Psychiatry 18:353–358, 2010

Guara A: Perceived coercion and change in perceived need for admission in patients hospitalized for eating disorders. Am J Psychiatry 164:108–114, 2007

Haidt J: The emotional dog and its rational tail: a social intuitionist approach to moral judgement. Psychol Rev 108(4):814–834, 2001

Harvard T.H. Chan School of Public Health: STRIPED: A Public Health Initiative. Mission and Rationale, 2019. Available at: https://www.hsph.harvard.edu/striped/introduction/mission-and-rationale. Accessed July 15, 2020.

Hudson JI, Hiripi E, Pope HG Jr, Kessler RC: The prevalence and correlates of eating disorders in the National Comorbidity Survey Replication. Biol Psychiatry 61(3):348–358, 2007

Johansson IM, Lundman B: Patients' experience of involuntary psychiatric care: good opportunities and great losses. J Psychiatr Ment Health Nurs 9(6):639–647, 2002

Kalvemark S, Höglund AT, Hansson MG, et al: Living with conflicts: ethical dilemmas and moral distress in the health care system. Soc Sci Med 58(6):1075–1084, 2004

Kendall S: Anorexia nervosa: the diagnosis. A postmodern ethics contribution to the bioethics debate on involuntary treatment for anorexia nervosa. J Bioeth Inq 11:31–40, 2014

Kontos N: Beyond capacity: identifying ethical dilemmas underlying capacity evaluation requests. Psychosomatics 54:103–110, 2013

Lauer CJ: Neuropsychological assessments before and after treatment in patients with anorexia nervosa and bulimia nervosa. J Psychiatr Res 33:129–138, 1999

Marques L, Alegria M, Becker AE, et al: Comparative prevalence, correlates of impairment, and service utilization for eating disorders across US ethnic groups: implications for reducing ethnic disparities in health care access for eating disorders. Int J Eat Disord 44(5): 412–420, 2011

Matusek JA, Wright MO: Ethical dilemmas in treating clients with eating disorders: a review and application of an integrative ethical decision-making model. Eur Eat Disord Rev 18:434–452, 2010

Medeiros GC: Anorexia nervosa, paternalism and clinical practice. Arch Clin Psychiatry 41(5):135, 2014

Montello M: Narrative ethics: the role of stories in bioethics, special report. The Hastings Center Report 44(1):S2–S6, 2014

Pellegrino E: The metamorphosis of medical ethics: a 30-year retrospective. JAMA 269(9):1158–1162, 1993

Pellegrino E, Thomasma D: The conflict between autonomy and beneficence in medical ethics: proposal for a resolution. J Contemp Health Law Policy 3(1):23–46, 1987

Sher Y, Sermsak L: Ethical issues: capacity to make medical decisions. Psychiatric Times 31(11), 2014

Singer PA, Pellegrino ED, Siegler M: Clinical ethics revised. BMC Med Ethics 2:1, 2001

Swanson JW: Facilitated psychiatric advance directives: a randomized trial of an intervention to foster advance treatment planning among persons with severe mental illness. Am J Psychiatry 163:1943–1951, 2006

Timmons M: Moral Theory: An Introduction, 2nd Edition. Lanham, MD, Rowman and Littlefield, 2013

Torke AM, Alexander GC, Lantos J: Substituted judgment: the limitations of autonomy in surrogate decision making. J Gen Intern Med 23(9):1514–1517, 2008

Traudt T: Moral agency, moral imagination, and moral community: antidotes to moral distress. J Clin Ethics 27(3):201–213, 2016

Túry F, Szalai T, Szumska I: Compulsory treatment in eating disorders: control, provocation, and the coercion paradox. J Clin Psychol 75(8):1444–1454, 2019

3

Coercion in Treatment

Angela S. Guarda, M.D.
Colleen C. Schreyer, Ph.D.

COERCIVE treatment has a long history in psychiatry and is controversial from clinical, legal, and ethical perspectives. Although often equated with compulsory treatment, coercive interventions occur along a spectrum ranging from gentle persuasion at one extreme to involuntary treatment at the other. Definitions of coercive treatment vary; however, a practical definition is that *coercive treatment* involves the infliction of physical or psychological distress by limiting a person's choice and autonomy, either by force or by a conditional threat (Szmukler 2015). Coercive pressure for treatment may be exerted through formal legal procedures as well as informally by clinicians, family members, or others concerned about the patient's welfare.

Coercion may further be distinguished as "objective" or "perceived." *Perceived coercion* reflects patients' beliefs about their ability to freely refuse treatment and may not be closely related to *objective coercion*, which may involve involuntary treatment, the use of chemical or physical restraints, or forced feeding (Opsal et al. 2016). Up to half of general psychiatric patients who are compulsorily admitted do not recognize their status as involuntary, whereas 30%–50% of patients admitted voluntarily feel they were coerced into the hospital or during their stay (Wynn 2006). Factors found to increase patients' perceptions of coercive treatment include 1) not feeling heard or having a say in treatment decisions, 2) not feeling that they are being treated respectfully, 3) not feeling sick enough to justify the intervention, 4) believing the treatment is unjust, or 5) not responding to treatment

(Monahan et al. 1995). We review the topic of coercion in the treatment of eating disorders (EDs) and cover relevant ethical principles, types of coercion, and the limited literature on the outcome of coercive interventions surrounding hospitalization and nutritional rehabilitation. We conclude with practical suggested guidelines to minimize coercion and its effects on the therapeutic alliance, as well as directions for future research.

Medical Ethics and Coercive Treatment

Balancing principles of medical ethics that often conflict with one another is one challenge in the treatment of severely ill psychiatric patients. These principles include respect for patient autonomy in decisions about care, nonmaleficence (the duty not to harm patients), beneficence (the duty to act in the best interest of the patient), and procedural justice (the fairness of a procedure or intervention). Ideally, treatment should minimize coercion, optimize clinical outcomes, and maximize patient satisfaction (Wynn 2006). Two of the most challenging ethical questions in the treatment of patients with anorexia nervosa (AN) are 1) When is involuntary hospitalization justified? and 2) When is it permissible to force feed a patient?

A relative consensus agrees that involuntary treatment is justified when psychiatric patients present an immediate danger to themselves or others, such as that acutely suicidal or homicidal patient. Controversy arises, however, when the risk is less clearly imminent, as often is the case with chronic and severe AN. Although AN has arguably the highest mortality among psychiatric conditions and is associated with elevated morbidity and functional impairment (Agh et al. 2016; Arcelus et al. 2011), imminent risk is difficult to assess. Judging when and how to optimally intervene in the care of a patient with life-threatening severe AN is challenging. Chronically ill patients may be unpredictably medically unstable, with their risk increasing and decreasing over a period of several years as their behavioral severity waxes and wanes. In addition, acute medical stabilization, such as correcting electrolytes in the emergency department, constitutes symptomatic treatment but does little to address the underlying state of starvation, mitigate risk, or treat the underlying psychiatric condition that led to the patient's presentation.

The use of legal coercion in the treatment of psychiatric patients may be justified when their decision-making ability regarding appropriate care is impaired by their illness, when the risk of death and disability is high, and when the likelihood of benefit from treatment is also high. This assumes that coercive treatment will restore decision-making capacity, alleviate suffering, and benefit the patient in the long term. Research on the effectiveness of coercion is challenging, however, and data are limited. Controlled trials are not ethically justified, and case control studies are biased because coerced samples have higher severity and lower treatment compliance or motivation to change. Despite these limitations, most studies of involuntary treatment in general psychiatric patients indicate that most view treatment as acceptable after the fact, although a minority do not, and in those for whom treatment was not successful, coercive interventions may result in future treatment avoidance (Swartz et al. 2003).

Eating Disorders as Motivated Behavioral Disorders: The Special Case of Anorexia Nervosa

EDs are driven behavioral disorders with parallels to addiction and are characterized by varying levels of ambivalence toward treatment and impairment of insight and decision making (Guarda 2008). Patients with severe EDs develop an increasingly constrained behavioral repertoire, stereotyped conditioned approach and avoidance behaviors to illness-related stimuli, and impaired choice over their actions. Over time, this leads to escalating disordered-eating and weight-control behaviors in the face of increasingly negative consequences. Despite the costs of the illness, patients often continue to provide seemingly rational explanations for their eating and weight-control behaviors, citing health concerns or personal values.

Among EDs, the most puzzling is AN, a syndrome of self-starvation. Evidence indicates that dysregulation of the neurocircuitry that underlie anxiety and reward and starvation-induced alterations in homeostatic hunger and satiety signaling contribute to maintenance of this disorder in genetically vulnerable individuals. Although most of these changes are state related and reverse with weight restoration, evidence suggests that some feed forward to sustain escalating restricting and exercise behaviors (Guarda 2008; Guarda et al. 2015). Additionally, AN is characterized by overvalued morbid eating restraint that develops into a zealously defended, consuming, and ego-syntonic passion. Ambivalence toward treatment aimed at weight gain or normalization of eating behavior can reach the level of treatment refusal and is a symptom of the disorder. Although their fear of fatness can appear near delusional in degree (Steinglass et al. 2007), patients maintain good reasoning in other areas. Most recognize a need to change their behavior but describe being of two minds, frequently viewing aspects of their illness positively, as part of their identity, and having difficulty imagining life without the disorder (Espindola and Blay 2009; Tan et al. 2003).

When individuals do seek treatment, they often do so on their own terms, picking and choosing recommendations that are less threatening to the core values of their illness. They prefer talk-based interventions that explore the "root cause" of the disorder over approaches that emphasize behavior change. Early behavior change is increasingly recognized as the primary transdiagnostic predictor of treatment response in EDs (MacDonald et al. 2017; Nazar et al. 2017). Recovery is a protracted process, however, that requires sustained normalization of eating and weight-control behaviors over time, reversal of the starved state, and improvements in psychological symptoms and functional status.

Importance of Weight Restoration in the Treatment of Anorexia Nervosa

Weight restoration is a necessary first step in recovery from AN, although about half of the patients who achieve this benchmark are at risk for relapse within 2 years (Berends et al. 2018). Despite this risk, a 22-year follow-up study found a 62% recovery rate. Furthermore, twice as many patients were recovered when assessed at 22 years compared with the 9-year assessment, suggesting that recovery is possible even in those with long-term, chronic AN (Eddy et al. 2017).

Effective treatments for AN are limited; however, in most adolescents with a short duration of illness, family-based outpatient treatment has been associated with a favorable prognosis (Lock and Le Grange 2018). For adults with AN, no outpatient intervention has yet proven effective in achieving weight restoration (Hay et al. 2015); however, expert consensus and correlational data support intensive hospital-based behavioral treatment for those who do not respond to outpatient care. A higher patient BMI at discharge from intensive treatment has been repeatedly associated with lower relapse and readmission rates (Kaplan et al. 2009; Rigaud et al. 2011; Sly and Bamford 2011), resulting in recent interest in improving the rates of weight restoration in these settings (Attia et al. 2017; Garber et al. 2016; Guarda et al. 2017).

Mean rates of weight gain in hospital-based treatment vary greatly by program and range from 0.5 kg/week to 2.0 kg/week (Friedman et al. 2016; Garber et al. 2016). With appropriate medical monitoring, rates of weight gain up to 2.0 kg/week have been found safe and appear tolerable even in very malnourished patients (Garber et al. 2016; Redgrave et al. 2015). No data link the rate of weight gain with increased perception of coercive treatment; the setting and the therapeutic rapport between the team and the patient, rather than the rate of weight gain or the prescribed calorie intake, are likely to be more closely predictive of patients' perceptions of the tolerability of a specific refeeding approach. Some medical stabilization and behavioral programs use supplemental tube feeding to boost lower rates of weight gain (Rizzo et al. 2019). Where used, nasogastric tube feeding may be protocol wide or only for patients who fail to meet their weekly weight-gain targets with meal-based feeding alone. Data comparing patient perceptions of meal-based feeding with those of enteral tube feeding approaches are lacking. Patient satisfaction with nasogastric feeds was only assessed in one study and did not differ between meal-based and enteral tube-fed patients; however, rates of weight gain in this study were low, averaging <1 kg/week (Zuercher et al. 2003). An argument has been made in favor of meal-based approaches over tube feeding whenever possible, both for safety reasons and because recovery requires the extinction of heightened meal-related anxiety about consuming various foods of differing caloric densities.

Informal Methods of Coercion

For patients with EDs, attempts to normalize weight and eating behavior feel threatening and contribute to treatment avoidance. Informal methods of social persuasion to seek care are therefore common and can come from family, friends, employers, educators, and clinicians in the form of coaxing, begging, bargaining, conditional threats, ultimatums, and providing selective information in order to induce patients to seek care. Besides influencing care seeking, informal methods of coercion are often central to effective behavioral interventions for EDs. In the treatment of adolescents with AN, for example, family-based treatment relies on the therapist empowering and training parents to take control of their child's meals by empathically and supportively insisting that food refusal and dieting are not an option and that food is medicine. The family-based therapist instructs parents to take control of portioning and preparing their child's food, supervising meals, and interrupting disordered behaviors until the child is able to manage his or her behavior in a healthy way (Stiles-Shields et al. 2012).

Because decisions about medical care for minors are generally made by parents or legal guardians, the treatment of minors with EDs is by nature more paternalistic. Consistent with the idea that adolescents are less free to refuse care, and despite having a more favorable prognosis than adults, hospitalized adolescents with EDs report higher levels of perceived coercion surrounding the admission process than do adults (Guarda et al. 2007; Hillen et al. 2015). Whether the better prognosis of adolescents is explained by a lower scar effect from chronic illness or by a less severe, self-limited form of the disorder is unclear in many cases. It is also possible that external parental involvement and leveraged treatment help interrupt disordered eating and weight-control behaviors, reverse the starved state, improve cognition and mood, and promote the formation of healthier eating habits.

Many adult patients with EDs also experience informal coercive pressure for admission. More patients with AN voluntarily hospitalized in an inpatient behavioral specialty program perceived their admission as coercive than did those with bulimia nervosa (BN), which is consistent with the more ego-syntonic nature of AN. One-third of the sample in this study reported that they did not need hospitalization at the time of admission and had been admitted under pressure from others. When perceived coercion and need for hospitalization were reassessed 2 weeks later, however, perceived coercion remained stable, but nearly half stated that they now recognized they had needed a higher level of care at the time they were admitted (Guarda et al. 2007). This shift in belief about the need for hospitalization may reflect clinicians' observation that as patients change their behavior and form a therapeutic alliance with the treatment team, their motivation to change improves (Guarda 2008). In another study, higher perceived coercion at admission in underweight patients with EDs was associated with higher drive for thinness and body dissatisfaction but did not impact hospital course or the likelihood of achieving weight restoration, although it did predict premature dropout following transition to a less supervised partial hospitalization program (Schreyer et al. 2016).

A significant body of research supports contingency management interventions for patients in addiction treatment (Cahill et al. 2015; Hartzler and Garrett 2016). In contrast, research examining contingency management strategies to encourage behavior change in patients with EDs is scarce. One systematic qualitative review suggested that enhancing the autonomy of patients with AN by encouraging their participation in drafting contingency contracts about their weekly weight gain expectations produced short-term favorable effects and may enhance their motivation, compliance, and sense of autonomy in treatment (Ziser et al. 2018a, 2018b). Furthermore, despite the lack of research in this area, elements of contingency management are inherent in intensive behavioral treatment programs for EDs (Matusek and Wright 2010). Most specialty programs employ a stepped-care protocol to help patients interrupt their eating and weight-control behaviors. Typical protocols include initial staff observation of meals and bathroom monitoring, as well as exercise restriction, with gradual transition to increased levels of independence. Additional common behavioral strategies that encourage the practice of healthier habits around food and exercise or meal completion but may be viewed by patients as restrictive of autonomy include limited visiting hours, locked units, redirection for disordered ritualistic table

behaviors such as smearing or dicing food or excessive movement, staff selection and portioning of food, provision of liquid supplements, and the
threat of nasogastric tube feeding if meals are not completed.

Formal Methods of Coercion

Formal coercion refers to using legal measures to compel treatment, including
involuntary hospitalization or outpatient commitment. Compulsory outpatient treatment for patients with severe mental illness has been justified as
a measure to help improve outcomes and reduce costs for high utilizers of
health care, but evidence for its impact on readmission rates, lengths of stay,
or treatment adherence remains unclear (Barnett et al. 2018). No current
studies have examined outpatient commitment procedures for patients with
EDs. Formal compulsory treatment for adults with EDs is therefore limited to involuntary hospitalization and primarily to studies on AN. Patients
with severe AN are more likely to be committed, either at hospital admission or when they seek to leave treatment prematurely, due to their elevated
mortality risk, need for prolonged hospitalization for renourishment, and
high frequency of treatment refusal. Although data on the frequency of involuntary hospitalization for AN are limited, a significant minority appear
to be involuntarily committed either at admission or during their hospital
stay, with rates as high as 40% in tertiary-referral behavioral specialty programs (Clausen and Jones 2014; Elzakkers et al. 2014).

Two systematic reviews summarized the existing literature in this area
(Clausen and Jones 2014; Elzakkers et al. 2014). Overall, involuntarily
treated patients with AN have more symptom severity and comorbidity,
more self-harm behaviors, more prior hospitalizations, and lower BMI at
admission. Their hospital course is notable for longer lengths of stay, and
they are more likely to be tube fed or treated on a locked unit than are voluntary patients. However, discharge BMI across studies does not differ between involuntary and voluntary patients, indicating short-term benefit and
success in weight restoration and reversal of the starved state. One long-
term follow-up case control study compared 81 voluntary and 81 involuntary patients treated in a specialty program in the United Kingdom and
found no group differences in standardized mortality rates at 20 years
(Ward et al. 2016).

Data indicating empirical harm from involuntary treatment are lacking. When effective, involuntary treatment is often met with gratitude by
patients and families, and formal complaints regarding its appropriateness
by patients are rare (Newton-Howes and Mullen 2011; Tiller et al. 1993;
Watson et al. 2000). Importantly, patients with AN have difficulty appreciating their own need for treatment, but most agree that, in principle, com-

pulsory treatment of others with the same condition is justified if needed to avoid death from AN (Tan et al. 2010). This ability to recognize the need for others to receive treatment is central to the effectiveness of group therapy approaches commonly employed in intensive treatment settings, where peer pressure is often a key factor in helping patients develop insight and increased motivation to change their behavior.

Formal coercion and involuntary hospitalization are tied to the assessment of the patient's capacity to consent to treatment. Involuntary treatment ethically requires that patients lack mental capacity to make decisions about their own care. Impaired capacity in AN is usually limited to the circumscribed area of agreeing to treatment likely to result in weight gain (Elzakkers et al. 2017, 2018). Indeed, qualitative data from patient interviews suggest that patients later recognize they had been unable to make their own decisions about care when at extremely low weights (Tan et al. 2010).

Effect of Coercion on the Treatment Alliance

For those who are involuntarily detained, the adversarial nature of the legal process can delay or interfere with forming a therapeutic alliance; however, this can also be the case with informal coercive interventions. Furthermore, the nature of AN itself challenges the therapeutic alliance, because patients often seek treatment on their own terms, not necessarily to change their behavior but to feel better, which puts the goals of patient and provider in conflict. Successful treatment requires a cognitive shift in the patient, akin to an ideological conversion, from viewing dieting as a solution to recognizing it as the problem.

To be effective, treatment must instill hope, win patients' cooperation, and help them move toward a tipping point at which motivation for recovery surpasses the pull of the ED (Dawson et al. 2014). Qualitative data from patient interviews suggest that trust in the patient–provider relationship is likely to moderate the experience of coercion in treatment (Tan et al. 2010). Perceived coercion is thus lower when the therapeutic relationship is strong and patients feel heard (Newton-Howes and Mullen 2011). Explaining the medical rationale for treatment decisions and respectfully and collaboratively including patients in team discussions may decrease feelings of powerlessness and alienation. Validating their ambivalence and demonstrating a caring and encouraging stance while acknowledging patients' struggle may help build rapport and trust. Patient role induction, including reviewing treatment goals and expectations for weight gain or behavior change, providing opportunities for exercising choice, and regularly assessing clinical progress, can be helpful. For hospitalized patients nearing discharge, drafting a written collaborative relapse-prevention or crisis plan stipulating criteria for rehospitalization may reduce the need for, or degree of, coercion during a future relapse (Szmukler 2015). Engagement of family members is also key to maximizing outcomes, and alignment between the family and the treatment team increases the likelihood of a patient's engagement and eventual conversion.

One study suggested the importance of an early therapeutic alliance in patients hospitalized with AN. Patients who rated their therapeutic alliance with their primary nurse highly were less likely to end their treatment early (Sly et al. 2013). Nursing staff in hospital-based specialty programs provide meal and bathroom supervision and play a pivotal role in patient engagement by encouraging patients to normalize their behavior and complete each meal. This work is challenging and requires psychotherapeutic skill, because patients often negotiate and bargain for exceptions to unit rules. Poorly compliant patients may engender countertransference in staff, including feelings of impotence or exasperation that challenge the therapeutic alliance. A setting of care, a supportive ward organization, staff training, and supervision are thought to be crucial elements of a program's success in maintaining a collaborative and therapeutic stance (Zugai et al. 2018).

Motivational interviewing strategies, including a focus on pro-recovery behaviors and support of self-efficacy to eat normally, aid in building rapport with reluctant patients. Although motivation-based interventions increase patients' motivation to change, evidence is mixed as to the effect of these strategies on treatment completion or clinically significant behavior change (Denison-Day et al. 2018; Sly et al. 2013). Of concern, perceived coercion is inversely related to motivation to change, and the prognostic value of stage of change has been associated with self-referral. This suggests that assessment of motivation to change may be complicated in coerced patients, because overreporting in an attempt to leave treatment earlier may be more common in this group. Although evidence is scarce, interventions that address motivation to change may be most effective for patients with higher baseline motivation who are closer to the action stage of change.

Conclusion

In the treatment of EDs, and especially with regard to AN, recognition is growing that some degree of coercion is inherent in most treatment interventions. Coercive measures range from gentle persuasion to involuntary treatment or nasogastric tube feeding. Clear evidence suggesting positive or negative consequences of coerced treatment is lacking, and further quantitative and qualitative research is needed to answer the complex ethical, clinical, and legal issues relevant to this topic. Future research should examine patient views on coercion in both voluntary and involuntary inpatient settings and in outpatient treatment samples, paying attention to the context of treatment delivery, treatment outcome, and predictors of a positive shift in therapeutic alliance among patients who experience their treatment as coercive. Systematic qualitative research examining patients' and family members' retrospective view of need for, and acceptability of, coercive treatment is also important for understanding the longer-term effects of coercive interventions. At minimum, we need data on the frequency that objective measures of coercion are used in the care of patients with EDs, including involuntary admission, physical or chemical restraints, and nasogastric forced feeding. Finally, research should explore methods to help reduce perceived coercion at the time of treatment admission by maximizing self-efficacy and self-determination for recovery. This information would benefit all stakeholders, including patients, family, providers, and insurers, as well as the legal system and policymakers.

References

Agh T, Kovacs G, Supina D, et al: A systematic review of the health-related quality of life and economic burdens of anorexia nervosa, bulimia nervosa, and binge eating disorder. Eat Weight Disord 21(3):353–364, 2016

Arcelus J, Mitchell AJ, Wales J, Nielsen S: Mortality rates in patients with anorexia nervosa and other eating disorders: a meta-analysis of 36 studies. Arch Gen Psychiatry 68(7):724–731, 2011

Attia E, Marcus MD, Walsh BT, Guarda AS: The need for consistent outcome measures in eating disorder treatment programs: a proposal for the field. Int J Eat Disord 50(3):231–234, 2017

Barnett P, Matthews H, Lloyd-Evans B, et al: Compulsory community treatment to reduce readmission to hospital and increase engagement with community care in people with mental illness: a systematic review and meta-analysis. Lancet Psychiatry 5(12):1013–1022, 2018

Berends T, Boonstra N, van Ellburg A: Relapse in anorexia nervosa: A systematic review and meta-analysis. Curr Opin Psychiary 31(6): 445-455, 2018

Cahill K, Hartmann-Boyce J, Perera R: Incentives for smoking cessation. Cochrane Database Syst Rev (5):CD004307, 2015

Clausen L, Jones AA: Systematic review of the frequency, duration, type and effect of involuntary treatment for people with anorexia nervosa, and an analysis of patient characteristics. J Eat Disord 2(1):29, 2014

Dawson L, Rhodes P, Touyz S: "Doing the impossible": the process of recovery from chronic anorexia nervosa. Qual Health Res 24(4):494–505, 2014

Denison-Day J, Appleton KM, Newell C, Muir S: Improving motivation to change amongst individuals with eating disorders: a systematic review. Int J Eat Disord 51(9):1033–1050, 2018

Eddy KT, Tabri N, Thomas JJ, et al: Recovery from anorexia nervosa and bulimia nervosa at 22-year follow-up. J Clin Psychiatry 78(2):184–189, 2017

Elzakkers I, Danner UN, Hoek HW, et al: Compulsory treatment in anorexia nervosa: a review. Int J Eat Disord 47(8):845–852, 2014

Elzakkers I, Danner UN, Sternheim LC, et al: Mental capacity to consent to treatment and the association with outcome: a longitudinal study in patients with anorexia nervosa. Br J Psychiatry Open 3(3):147–153, 2017

Elzakkers I, Danner UN, Grisso T, et al: Assessment of mental capacity to consent to treatment in anorexia nervosa: a comparison of clinical judgment and MacCAT-T and consequences for clinical practice. Int J Law Psychiatry 58:27–35, 2018

Espindola CR, Blay SL: Anorexia nervosa's meaning to patients: a qualitative synthesis. Psychopathology 42(2):69–80, 2009

Friedman K, Ramirez AL, Murray SB, et al: A narrative review of outcome studies for residential and partial hospital-based treatment of eating disorders. Eur Eat Disord Rev 24(4):263–276, 2016

Garber AK, Sawyer SM, Golden NH, et al: A systematic review of approaches to refeeding in patients with anorexia nervosa. Int J Eat Disord 49(3):293–310, 2016

Guarda AS: Treatment of anorexia nervosa: insights and obstacles. Physiol Behav 94(1):113–120, 2008

Guarda AS, Pinto AM, Coughlin JW, et al: Perceived coercion and change in perceived need for admission in patients hospitalized for eating disorders. Am J Psychiatry 164(1):108–114, 2007

Guarda AS, Schreyer CC, Boersma GJ, et al: Anorexia nervosa as a motivated behavior: relevance of anxiety, stress, fear and learning. Physiol Behav 152(pt B):466–472, 2015

Guarda AS, Schreyer CC, Fischer LK, et al: Intensive treatment for adults with anorexia nervosa: the cost of weight restoration. Int J Eat Disord 50(3):302–306, 2017

Hartzler B, Garrett S: Interest and preferences for contingency management design among addiction treatment clientele. Am J Drug Alcohol Abuse 42(3):287–295, 2016

Hay PJ, Claudino AM, Touyz S, Abd Elbaky G: Individual psychological therapy in the outpatient treatment of adults with anorexia nervosa. Cochrane Database Syst Rev (7):CD003909, 2015

Hillen S, Dempfle A, Seitz J, et al: Motivation to change and perceptions of the admission process with respect to outcome in adolescent anorexia nervosa. BMC Psychiatry 15:140, 2015

Kaplan AS, Walsh BT, Olmsted M, et al: The slippery slope: prediction of successful weight maintenance in anorexia nervosa. Psychol Med 39(6):1037–1045, 2009

Lock J, Le Grange D: Family based treatment: where are we and where should we be going to improve recovery in child and adolescent eating disorders. Int J Eat Disord 52(4):481–487, 2018

MacDonald DE, McFarlane TL, Dionne MM, et al: Rapid response to intensive treatment for bulimia nervosa and purging disorder: a randomized controlled trial of a CBT intervention to facilitate early behavior change. J Consult Clin Psychol 85(9):896–908, 2017

Matusek JA, Wright MO: Ethical dilemmas in treating clients with eating disorders: a review and application of an integrative ethical decision-making model. Eur Eat Disord Rev 18(6):434–452, 2010

Monahan J, Hoge SK, Lidz C, et al: Coercion and commitment: understanding involuntary mental hospital admission. Int J Law Psychiatry 18(3):249–263, 1995

Nazar BP, Gregor LK, Albano G, et al: Early response to treatment in eating disorders: a systematic review and a diagnostic test accuracy meta-analysis. Eur Eat Disord Rev 25(2):67–79, 2017

Newton-Howes G, Mullen R: Coercion in psychiatric care: systematic review of correlates and themes. Psychiatr Serv 62(5):465–470, 2011

Opsal A, Kristensen O, Vederhus JK, Clausen T: Perceived coercion to enter treatment among involuntarily and voluntarily admitted patients with substance use disorders. BMC Health Serv Res 16(1):656, 2016

Redgrave GW, Coughlin JW, Schreyer CC, et al: Refeeding and weight restoration outcomes in anorexia nervosa: challenging current guidelines. Int J Eat Disord 48(7):866–873, 2015

Rigaud D, Pennacchio H, Bizeul C, et al: Outcome in AN adult patients: a 13-year follow-up in 484 patients. Diabetes Metab 37(4):305–311, 2011

Rizzo SM, Douglas JW, Lawrence JC: Enteral nutrition via nasogastric tube for refeeding patients with anorexia nervosa: a systematic review. Nutr Clin Pract 34(3):359–370, 2019

Schreyer CC, Coughlin JW, Makhzoumi SH, et al: Perceived coercion in inpatients with anorexia nervosa: associations with illness severity and hospital course. Int J Eat Disord 49(4):407–412, 2016

Sly R, Bamford B: Why are we waiting? The relationship between low admission weight and end of treatment weight outcomes. Eur Eat Disord Rev 19(5):407–410, 2011

Sly R, Morgan JF, Mountford VA, Lacey JH: Predicting premature termination of hospitalised treatment for anorexia nervosa: the roles of therapeutic alliance, motivation, and behaviour change. Eat Behav 14(2):119–123, 2013

Steinglass JE, Eisen JL, Attia E, et al: Is anorexia nervosa a delusional disorder? An assessment of eating beliefs in anorexia nervosa. J Psychiatr Pract 13(2):65–71, 2007

Stiles-Shields C, Hoste RR, Doyle PM, Le Grange D: A review of family based treatment for adolescents with eating disorders. Rev Recent Clin Trials 7(2):133–140, 2012

Swartz MS, Swanson JW, Hannon MJ: Does fear of coercion keep people away from mental health treatment? Evidence from a survey of persons with schizophrenia and mental health professionals. Behav Sci Law 21(4):459–472, 2003

Szmukler G: Compulsion and "coercion" in mental health care. World Psychiatry 14(3):259–261, 2015

Tan J, Hope T, Stewart A: Competence to refuse treatment in anorexia nervosa. Int J Law Psychiatry 26(6):697–707, 2003

Tan J, Stewart A, Fitzpatrick R, Hope T: Attitudes of patients with anorexia nervosa to compulsory treatment and coercion. Int J Law Psychiatry 33(1):13–19, 2010

Tiller J, Schmidt U, Treasure J: Compulsory treatment for anorexia nervosa: compassion or coercion? Br J Psychiatry 162:679–680, 1993

Ward A, Ramsay R, Russell G, Treasure J: Follow-up mortality study of compulsorily treated patients with anorexia nervosa. Int J Eat Disord 49(4):435, 2016

Watson TL, Bowers WA, Andersen AE: Involuntary treatment of eating disorders. Am J Psychiatry 157(11):1806–1810, 2000

Wynn R: Coercion in psychiatric care: clinical, legal, and ethical controversies. Int J Psychiatry Clin Pract 10(4):247–251, 2006

Ziser K, Giel KE, Resmark G, et al: Contingency contracts for weight gain of patients with anorexia nervosa in inpatient therapy: practice styles of specialized centers. J Clin Med 7(8):215, 2018a

Ziser K, Resmark G, Giel KE, et al: The effectiveness of contingency management in the treatment of patients with anorexia nervosa: a systematic review. Eur Eat Disord Rev 26(5):379–393, 2018b

Zuercher JN, Cumella EJ, Woods BK, et al: Efficacy of voluntary nasogastric tube feeding in female inpatients with anorexia nervosa. JPEN 27(4):268–276, 2003

Zugai JS, Stein-Parbury J, Roche M: Therapeutic alliance, anorexia nervosa and the inpatient setting: a mixed methods study. J Adv Nurs 74(2):443–453, 2018

4

Mental Capacity in Anorexia Nervosa

Isis Elzakkers, M.D., Ph.D.
Cushla McKinney, Ph.D., M.B.H.L.

What Is Mental Capacity?

Current medicolegal practice recognizes the absolute right of individuals to make their own decisions regarding whether to accept or reject treatment unless there is reason to believe that their autonomy is compromised. This position is grounded in the idea that patients, rather than physicians, are in the best position to judge their own best interests and that freedom of choice is necessary for—or more important than—ensuring their physical welfare. Autonomous decisions are those made competently (with full and rational consideration of all relevant information) and voluntarily (free from undue influence). *Competence* and *capacity* are often used interchangeably, and their exact definitions vary by country and jurisdiction (legal or medical)[1], but as generally understood, *mental capacity* relates to a person's

---

[1]How medical and psychiatric patients are assessed also may differ, and ethical arguments can be made for aligning the criteria for competence and capacity because of the potential for differential outcomes depending on whether the patient is assessed for involuntary treatment under civil or mental health legislation (see, e.g., Owen et al. 2013 and Tan and McMillan 2004).

cognitive ability to understand the nature and effects of his or her actions and decisions relative to a normative standard (Applebaum and Grisso 1988; Beauchamp and Childress 1979; Buchanan and Brock 1989; summarized by Charland 2015).

Because people's ability to make free and reasoned choices about their own lives is considered a prerequisite for autonomous action, tests of capacity are used as a way to measure a person's ability to

- Understand and retain information relevant to the question at hand
- Comprehend that information in relation to their own circumstances (appreciation)
- Weigh the pros and cons of the information and make a decision (reasoning)
- Communicate that decision

General Principles

Patients are considered to have mental capacity unless one has reason to think otherwise. An unwise or eccentric decision is not necessarily an indication of lack of capacity, because what people consider to be in their own best interest can extend beyond what benefits them medically; they may have other values and preferences, and we allow people to make all sorts of irrational or apparently unreasonable decisions about treatment (including refusing life-sustaining intervention) because we respect their beliefs and desires. For example, a patient with a potentially curable cancer might reject chemotherapy in favor of palliative care because he or she would rather have a reasonable quality of life for whatever time remains than experience the consequences of an aggressive treatment with no guarantee of success. Illness is, for that patient, one episode in the ongoing narrative of life, and any consideration of benefit needs to incorporate both the patient's own views about the type of life he or she wishes to live and the patient's subjective experience of both illness and treatment. Thus, the decision-making *process*, not the outcome, is the critical factor in deciding whether it is ethically (and legally) permissible to override a person's wishes (Buchanan and Brock 1989; Freedman 1981). Provided the patient's choice is made freely and with adequate information, neither the *content* of those wishes and desires nor the subsequent *outcome* are material to determining autonomy. We assess capacity on procedural terms rather than whether we consider the final outcome sensible or normal.

Patients' ability to make choices depends on the nature of the decision they are making and the context in which they make it. It is also influenced by a variety of intrinsic and extrinsic factors and may fluctuate over time. However, we assume that everyone has the capacity to make their own decisions if given enough information, support, and time. As much as possible, clinicians must provide a supportive environment that minimizes the possibility of external influences undermining patients' mental capacity.

Incapacity is decision specific and may be global or local. Individuals may not be able to make reasoned decisions in relation to certain treatment decisions because their cognitive ability is impaired by illness, but they retain capacity in relation to choices (e.g., whether to accept or refuse tests or treatment for minor or unrelated physical conditions) or judgments related to other aspects of their life (Buchanan and Brock 1989). In general, the level of capacity required to make an informed decision also depends on the complexity and gravity of the situation. The greater the level of understanding required and the more serious the consequences, the higher the threshold for capacity, although this is still the subject of some dispute (Cale 1999; den Hartogh 2016).

When to Consider Assessment

Because decision-making capacity is specific to a particular situation and can vary over time as a person's condition and circumstances change, it should be assessed every time a medical decision is necessary. As a general rule, we presume people have the capacity to make treatment decisions unless we have reason to question their cognitive ability. This could include both formal thought disorders, such as psychoses, and circumstances in which their lack of insight and impaired judgment has left them unable to appreciate the life-threatening consequences of refusing treatment (Applebaum and Grisso 1988). Situations that may compromise a patient's capacity include traumatic head injury, psychosis, dementia, delirium, the effects of therapeutic or recreational drugs, intoxication, and severe mental retardation. A patient's mental capacity might also be questioned if the decision being made is likely to lead to serious and preventable harm, but this must be linked to an underlying psychopathology rather than a particular worldview; a formal assessment of capacity is most frequently carried out when patients refuse treatment. This distinction is particularly important in the context of psychiatric illness; although we may tend to assume that the illness in and of itself leads to incapacity, most psychiatric patients retain the capacity to make reasoned decisions (Candia and Barba 2011). Individuals with mental illness may also be under considerable pressure from friends, family, and medical and psychiatric professionals to undertake "voluntary" treatment. Although we require patients to give informed consent before any medical procedure is carried out, we assume that the treatment is in their best interest.

Capacity, and an individual's goals, preferences, and values, can fluctuate over time. When patients undergo extended periods of treatment, their capacity should be regularly reassessed to account for changes in their condition and circumstances. This may be problematic if a patient frequently changes his or her viewpoint. If the patient's inability to reach a settled decision prevents the effective implementation of care, this could be regarded as a sign of incapacity (Applebaum and Grisso 1988).

Effects of Nutrition on Capacity

Starvation often leads to depression and, in extreme cases, delusions (fixed false beliefs). Even in people who are otherwise healthy, extended restriction of food intake will lead to poor concentration and slow and muddled thinking. Although a systematic study of the effects of short-term fasting was equivocal on the impact of hunger on general cognition (Benau et al. 2014), other starvation-related changes observed in AN, such as reduced cognitive flexibility, have also have been reported in healthy people who fast on a short-term basis (Piech et al. 2009). Extended periods of starvation also result in other symptoms characteristic of AN. Concentration camp survivors and research subjects in food-restriction experiments develop intense preoccupations with food, heightened emotional responsiveness (particularly irritability and negative emotionality), cognitive disturbances such as obsessive rumination about food, narcissism and infantile regression, and loss of interest in other areas of life (Keys et al. 1950). These changes occur as a result of their physical state rather than being characteristic of AN, per se, and can be resolved with weight gain. However, even in healthy people, symptoms such as food obsessions, a loss of control around food, and episodes of binge eating can persist after weight is restored (Polivy 1996).

Other characteristics, such as the way hunger is experienced, denial of physical weakness, and pride in weight loss seem to be unique to AN (Bruch 1978). Rapid reduction in cognitive symptoms related to starvation, such as food preoccupation, irritability, mood swings, and apathy, has been noted to occur within the first 4 weeks of refeeding, prior to any significant change in BMI (Calugi et al. 2018). Interestingly, in this study, a positive correlation was found between the rate of symptom resolution, overall improvement in Eating Disorder Examination score, and reduction in weight concerns and general psychopathology, both at the end of the treatment period and at 6-month posttreatment follow-up, suggesting that starvation reinforces eating disorder (ED) behaviors, such as rigidity and anxiety, that may make people less able to change their behavior (Calugi et al. 2018).

In addition to the profound endocrine changes that occur in severe AN (reviewed in Støving 2019), studies of brain structure, blood flow, and neurological functioning in underweight and recovered/weight-restored patients with AN have identified changes in frontal, limbic, occipital, striatal, and cerebellar regions involved in various neurological pathways and aspects of cognitive functioning. These include reward, emotional processing, and learning circuitry. Although more research is needed to distinguish between the physiological symptoms of starvation and those specific to AN (Hay and Sachdev 2011; Phillipou et al. 2018), some changes induced by starvation are only partially ameliorated by weight restoration (Lao-Kaim et al. 2015; Phillipou et al. 2014; Tchanturia et al. 2004). This may be because these features are trait dependent rather than state dependent. Changes in brain structure and function not resolved by weight gain may result from the physiological effects of caloric restriction combined with an individual's brain structure or physiology. Such variations in brain structure and function may depend on genetic factors, and several large-scale studies looking for genetic loci associated with AN have been carried out or are under way (reviewed in Baker et al. 2017). To date, six loci with a genome-wide level of significance have been identified, and evidence suggests that some genetic variants influencing schizophrenia and BMI may also contribute to susceptibility to AN, although these results have yet to be replicated.

Assessing Capacity in Patients With Severe Eating Disorders

As previously noted, to be considered to have adequate mental capacity, patients must understand, appreciate, and evaluate a medical situation and the treatments offered and be able to choose between options (Appelbaum and Roth 1982; Roth et al. 1977). To assess whether they are able to understand, appreciate, evaluate, and choose, physicians must clearly explain the situation to them. This may seem obvious, but research has shown that it does not always occur, and explaining an illness and its treatment more carefully and thoroughly can improve a patient's mental capacity (Carpenter et al. 2000; Lapid et al. 2003, 2004). If the information has not been explained adequately, one cannot conclude the person has inadequate decisional capacity, only that the clinician has given inadequate information on which to base that decision. Evaluators must clearly explain the degree of illness and, rather than belittle patients when they have another view of the medical situation, calmly discuss their perspective. People have the right to disagree with the evaluators. Evaluators must also discuss what treatment is advised; for a person contemplating ED treatment, it is important to explain what treatment will mean in terms of hospital stay (e.g., 24-hour, partial hospitalization, outpatient care), advised food intake, weight goal, and time commitment (e.g., ability to attend work/school, time away from home and family). It is also important to explain the expected goals of treatment, not only with regard to medical progress but also for improving psychological issues (e.g., depression, anxiety, obsessive-compulsive behaviors). Alternative treatments and the option of refusing treatment should also be explained. Transparency is paramount, and the risks and benefits of treatment versus no treatment should be made clear. Predicting what will happen as a result of choosing treatment or no treatment is often fraught with difficulty. However, as a result of their experience and medical knowledge, evaluators should be able to fully discuss with patients what may occur as a result of choosing various forms of treatment or no treatment at all.

If a decision regarding medical care is not acutely necessary, patients should take time to consider the decision, consulting family and friends as needed. Obviously, when a person overtly denies being ill at all, or denies the existence of a severe medical situation, it is likely he or she will be assessed as not having adequate decision-making capacity. However, the outcome is often not that clear. Patients with a severe ED might acknowledge being ill, even severely ill, but not believe the illness to be as severe as the treating physician or evaluator advises. They might acknowledge that the proposed treatment may benefit other patients with AN but believe it is not applicable in their case. They may advocate for other forms of treatment, some of which may or may not be appropriate, and the evaluator must assess whether the proposed alternative treatment has any merit.

The most complex assessments are those in which the patient verbally displays understanding, appreciation, and adequate reasoning but the evaluator has a "gut feeling" that what the patient says is not what the patient really believes. Knowing the person's history, background, and future aspirations helps when dealing with this difficult situation. Conferring with colleagues might also shed more light on how to deal with this particular assessment and set of circumstances.

The evaluator should prepare for the interview with the person whose capacity is in question by considering nuances particular to individuals with EDs. Several elements are pertinent in this regard:

1. Characteristics of the individual:

   a. *Stage of the illness*: The person may be in the early stages of an ED or may have had the illness for many years. In addition, the illness may be severe and imminently life threatening or less severe. The longer the duration of illness, the less likely the patient will achieve full remission (Steinhausen 2002). Alternately, the shorter the duration of and less severe the illness, the more likely the person will be able to recover fully.

b. *Treatment history*: If the person has successfully engaged in treatment in the past and had one or more periods of remission, it is more likely he or she will benefit from further treatment. If treatment has not led to improvement or periods of remission in the past, or if prior involuntary treatment has not been successful, future attempts at a full course of treatment should be approached cautiously.

c. *Comorbid psychiatric disorders*: Evaluators should assess whether any comorbid disorders, such as depression, anxiety, OCD, PTSD, autism spectrum disorder, personality disorder, or substance use disorders, are contributing to the individual's mental capacity issues.

d. *Motivation for treatment*: Some patients are very motivated, whereas others are ambivalent or amotivated. If the person has no motivation for treatment, it is highly likely that he or she will offer strong resistance and experience forced or coerced treatment as traumatic. The capacity evaluator also must pay attention to the possible contribution of comorbid disorders and their effect on motivation and assess why the person developed an ED; for example, AN sometimes develops from a desire to be thin, but being abnormally thin then becomes that person's identity, lowering his or her motivation to change behavior. The feeling of numbness associated with starvation may also be used to cope with trauma or assuage anxiety related to adult life.

2. Situational characteristics:

a. *Medical situation*: How severe is the patient's current medical condition? The more severe the condition and the higher the risk of death, the higher the threshold for mental capacity. Although this variable threshold is debatable because it may introduce arbitrariness in assessments (DeMarco 2002), it is a clinically logical course of action (Hotopf 2005).

b. *Emergency status*: Is there time to consider alternative treatment options or delay decisions regarding treatment, or is immediate action required?

c. *Family*: What is the family's opinion regarding the patient's course of illness, experience with his or her willingness to seek treatment, and their opinion of possible involuntary treatment? Consider also the family's relationship with the patient and their own burden of illness (e.g., resentment and anger toward the patient, caregiver fatigue).

d. *Treatment characteristics*: What treatment is advised? Are accessible and appropriate treatments available? Does the patient require hospitalization on a medical unit prior to being treated on a psychiatric inpatient unit? Is there an appropriate vertically integrated program offering inpatient or residential treatment, followed by partial hospitalization? If involuntary treatment is being considered, does the treatment team have sufficient experience with involuntary treatment? Is there even a treatment facility where involuntary treatment is available?

Clinical Interview Versus Quantitative Assessment

Mental capacity is usually assessed in a patient interview. However, interrater reliability has been shown to be low, and mental capacity is often overestimated (Kitamura and Kitamura 2000; Lepping 2011; Lepping et al. 2010; Marson et al. 1997; Shah and Mukherjee 2003; Vellinga et al. 2004). Thus, a semistructured interview was developed with the goal of standardizing capacity assessments. The work of Appelbaum and Grisso formed the basis of this assessment tool, the MacArthur Competence Assessment Tool for Treatment (MacCAT-T; Grisso et al. 1997). The MacCAT-T provides ratings for four subscales: Understanding (0–6), Appreciation (0–4), Reasoning (0–8), and Choice (0–2). It has been used in a wide range of medical and psychiatric situations and consistently demonstrates high interrater reliability (Candia and Barba 2011; Okai et al. 2007; Wang et al. 2017); it has therefore become the instrument of choice for scientific research into mental capacity. In clinical practice, however, it is not yet in wide use.

Research into the mental capacity of patients with severe EDs is surprisingly scarce considering the complex nature of the concept and the discussion regarding mental capacity in AN. Patients often show resistance to treatment and seem to behave irrationally, especially in light of the severe consequences of their illness. One of these seemingly irrational behaviors is reflected in the fact that only a minority of patients are treated within the mental health care system (Hoek 2006; Keski-Rahkonen et al. 2007; Smink et al. 2012).

In general psychiatry, a range of studies has examined mental capacity, and two reviews (Candia and Barba 2011; Okai et al. 2007) and one meta-analysis (Wang et al. 2017) have been published. Most use the MacCAT-T to assess capacity. Schizophrenia, bipolar disorder, and major depressive disorder were the most common diagnoses in the two reviews, but the meta-analysis studied only patients with schizophrenia. Psychosis, symptom severity, involuntary admission, and treatment refusal were indicators of incapacity. Okai et al. (2007) found that 29% of patients lacked capacity, and Wang et al. (2017) found that patients performed worse than healthy control subjects on all MacCAT-T subscales. The MacCAT-T significantly and persistently raises the proportion of patients found to have diminished mental capacity compared with clinical interview alone (Cairns et al. 2005; Vollmann et al. 2003); for instance, in patients with major depressive disorder, the proportion with diminished mental capacity was 3% according to clinicians but 20% on the MacCAT-T. For patients with schizophrenia, these numbers were 18% and 53%, respectively (Vollmann et al. 2003). Owen et al. (2013) compared mental capacity in physically ill and psychiatrically ill patients and noted that when physically ill patients have diminished capacity, it is mainly their reasoning that is deficient, whereas in psychiatrically ill patients with diminished capacity, their ability to appreciate the consequences of their decisions is most affected.

In patients with AN, only three clinical studies have been published to date, two in adolescent populations and one in adults. One small qualitative study (Tan et al. 2003b) using the MacCAT-T did not show any problems in capacity to consent to treatment among a sample of 10 adolescents with severe AN. Another qualitative study of 35 adolescents with AN also used the MacCAT-T (Turrell et al. 2011) and found mild problems with reasoning for patients with AN compared with healthy control subjects. In a study in adults (Elzakkers et al. 2016), one-third of 70 adult patients with a mean BMI of 15.5 kg/m^2 had diminished mental capacity at baseline, a remarkably high proportion compared with studies of mental capacity in other psychiatric populations. Diminished capacity was associated with a lower BMI, reduced appreciation of the degree of illness and need for treatment (as measured by the Mac-CAT-T), previous treatment for AN, low social functioning, and poor set shifting. The duration of illness did not differ between the groups. Patients had a range of comorbid psychiatric disorders (mainly depressive disorder and PTSD), but these were not associated with diminished mental capacity. Although BMI was significantly different between the two groups in this study, 43% of patients with a BMI <15 kg/m^2 were assessed to have mental capacity, highlighting the importance of looking further than BMI alone when assessing a patient's capacity to consent to treatment in AN. Importantly, almost all patients (92%) followed the advice given by professionals regarding treatment, suggesting that the acceptance of treatment-related advice does not necessarily indicate full mental capacity.

Taken together, the results of these studies show that patients with AN are likely at risk for diminished mental capacity, although further studies need to be done. Clinicians treating patients with AN have long since believed that mental capacity might be hampered in these patients, especially those who are severely underweight. These studies provide at least some science to support that clinical intuition. Patients with a very low BMI who have been treated previously for their AN, function poorly in society, and do not fully appreciate that they are severely ill have a higher likelihood of diminished mental capacity. In such patients, it is even more important to discuss treatment options when dealing with resistance.

Longitudinal studies are important for determining whether patients with diminished mental capacity have a different course of illness or poorer prognosis. To date, only one such study has been completed (Elzakkers et al. 2017); in this study, prognosis was more unfavorable for the group with diminished mental capacity to consent to treatment. After a 2-year follow-up period, patients with full capacity had, on average, mild AN, whereas those with diminished mental capacity still fell in the moderately ill category according to DSM-5 (American Psychiatric Association 2013). In the group with diminished mental capacity, more than half of patients (54%) had not achieved remission after 2 years, whereas in the group that did not lack capacity, only 27% had not achieved remission. In addition, those with diminished mental capacity demonstrated a higher likelihood of requiring inpatient treatment during those 2 years. Although the group with diminished capacity had a lower BMI at baseline, other parameters of prognostic relevance, such as duration of illness or the percentage of patients with the purging subtype of AN or comorbid diagnoses, were equal between groups. These findings suggest a longer duration of care and a more unfavorable prognosis for those with diminished mental capacity.

Next to the more obvious factor of BMI, diminished capacity seems to be a factor of relevance to prognosis. However, the means by which capacity impacts prognosis remains unclear. A possible precursor of diminished capacity may lie in the less adaptive decision making often demonstrated by patients with AN (Cavedini et al. 2006; Danner et al. 2016; Tchanturia et al. 2007; Wu et al. 2016). Decision making is a complex neuropsychological process in which several factors play a role. One such factor is reward. Interestingly, patients with AN view food restriction as rewarding (Decker et al. 2015; Fairburn et al. 1999; Fladung et al. 2010; Kaye et al. 2013; Keating 2010; Shafran and de Silva 2005; Zink and Weinberger 2010). This remarkable feature of AN seems counterintuitive to healthy people, but people with AN value food restriction, being thin, and exercising over almost anything else. Research suggests that state-dependent abnormalities in reward and decision-making regions inform the learning process and that this is how food restriction becomes a habitual choice over time (Decker et al. 2015; Foerde et al. 2015; Wu et al. 2016). Cavedini et al. (2006) showed that patients with AN who had maladaptive decision making gained less weight than patients with adaptive decision making. They suggested that this less adaptive decision making may interfere with the person's ability to profit from treatment. A further study assessing mental capacity in patients with AN showed that decision making was more maladaptive in patients with diminished mental capacity and that this was independent of BMI, the level of depression, and alexithymia (Elzakkers et al. 2016). Moreover, these decision-making deficiencies did not disappear with weight improvement (Elzakkers et al. 2017).

In summary, maladaptive decision making and aberrant reward processing are recognized in AN. These may be more hampered in people with diminished mental capacity, leading to a lesser degree of appreciation of their illness and a poor ability to benefit from treatment. However, this is all tentative, and further research is needed.

Assessment Challenges in Patients With Severe Eating Disorders

Too Much Focus on Cognitive Factors

The mental capacity assessment itself is often criticized as focusing too much on cognitive and rational functioning (Breden and Vollmann 2004; Charland 1998), although decision making is not wholly rational but rather is greatly influenced by emotional factors (Naqvi et al. 2006). When making complex decisions, individuals must rely on intuition as well as rational functioning, because our working memory capacity (and therefore cognitive capacity) is limited (Remmers and Michalak 2016). Adaptive decision making entails relying on intuition—that is, feelings or bodily signals, often referred to as *somatic markers* (Damasio 1994, 1996). Somatic markers result from the decision-making process when evaluative feedback (e.g., reward vs. punishment) is received and will bias decision making in an adaptive direction. However, disturbances in the affective system can hamper the reliance on these bodily feelings, and the decision-making process will likely be less adaptive.

In AN, some have expressed concern that mental capacity assessments focus too much on cognitive ability and too little on emotions (Breden and Vollmann 2004; Charland 1998, 2007; Tan 2003; Tan et al. 2006, 2009; Vollmann 2006). In patients with AN, psychiatric comorbidity occurs more often than not; mood disorders occur in nearly 75% and anxiety disorders in 25%–75% (Fernandez-Aranda et al. 2007; Raney et al. 2008). Although it is tempting to presume a connection between affective disturbances and diminished mental capacity, this has not yet been confirmed (Elzakkers et al. 2017). In this study, Elzakkers et al. (2017) suggested that a relative inability to regulate emotions was more likely to be related to capacity than to negative affect.

Whose Values Are Being Considered?

Another major point of criticism in the assessment of capacity in AN is that patients' values do not get enough merit in the MacCAT-T. Altered values (so-called pathological values) toward life and death have been noted in patients with current AN compared with those who have recovered (Tan et al. 2003b, 2003c). Tan et al. (2003a) also noted, in qualitative studies, that AN often becomes part of the person's personal identity, in contrast to other mental disorders (e.g., anxiety or depression) that patients see as separate entities. Because of the profound way AN can influence a person's beliefs and values, there is doubt as to whether mental capacity assessments can grasp the subtleties of such issues in this condition.

Sturman (2005) suggested that the distorted or false beliefs commonly encountered in patients with AN may not emerge well enough in the mental capacity assessment even though they have a profound impact on patients' choices. Grisso and Appelbaum (2006), authors of the MacCAT-T, remarked in response that the assessment of appreciation in that measure captures the effect of emotion and personal values. In addition, they warned against complicating the concept of mental capacity by adding the element of pathological values. They opined that the sensitivity and reliability of the assessment might be compromised, and individuals' rights diminished, by using such a moral concept. In the study by Elzakkers et al. (2016), *appreciation* was diminished, not the other abilities of the mental capacity assessment. This speaks in favor of the MacCAT-T's ability to capture at least part of these pathological values. However, although appreciation was diminished, this was subtle and by no means as obvious as in other psychiatric disorders (Vollmann et al. 2003).

A review of studies in patients with depression in which appreciation was also diminished in the mental capacity assessment suggested that impaired appreciation could compromise capacity in two ways: 1) inability to appreciate future possibilities as a result of affective symptoms distorting or blinding individuals' perception of the future, and 2) inability to maintain a minimal concern for the self (Hindmarch et al. 2013). These features have also been noted in individuals with AN.

In summary, the discussion regarding appreciation and values is not yet resolved. Values are just as important in decision making (and hence mental capacity). However, impairments in mental capacity appear to be more subtle in AN than in other psychiatric disorders, which suggests that the assessment of capacity to consent to treatment might be even more complex than in other psychiatric disorders.

Clinical Judgment vs. the MacCAT-T

As mentioned earlier, mental capacity can be assessed using clinical judgment or the MacCAT-T. In most psychiatric disorders, the proportion of patients found to lack capacity rises significantly when the MacCAT-T is used instead of or in conjunction with clinical judgment (Cairns et al. 2005; Vollmann et al. 2003). Clinical judgment is often unreliable, and capacity is overestimated (Kitamura and Kitamura 2000; Lepping 2011; Lepping et al. 2010; Marson et al. 1997; Shah and Mukherjee 2003; Vellinga et al. 2004); thus, one can argue that mental capacity assessments should be performed using the MacCAT-T. However, although seen as the gold standard in research, the MacCAT-T is not yet widely used in clinical practice. Part of the explanation for this might be that the results of scientific research trickle down to clinical reality rather slowly. Another explanation is that discussion regarding the MacCAT-T's ability to actually grasp what is important in mental capacity is not yet resolved. Although it has demonstrated superior interrater reliability, this does not necessarily mean that it is the more valid assessment. Because clinical assessments involve a degree of subjectivity, one may be tempted to look for an objective, quantifiable method for determining mental capacity. However, capacity is a concept with complex ethical, moral, and philosophical dimensions not easily captured by an image or a laboratory result, which argues against a purely scientific assessment approach.

In AN, the marked disagreement between the two forms of assessment reflects this tension. Both assessments (clinical judgment and MacCAT-T) found that one-third of patients had diminished mental capacity, but agreement between these two assessments was rather low (Elzakkers et al. 2018). Even capacity assessments of patients with schizophrenia and depression have not led to as many being deemed incapacitated. Clearly, the use of the MacCAT-T in AN encounters specific issues not seen in other psychiatric disorders. The claim that it emphasizes cognitive abilities and is less sensitive to values or emotions might, in part, explain the difference between the clinical evaluation and the semistructured assessment tool. In AN, emotional dysregulation (difficulty in recognizing and processing emotions) is a well-known maintaining factor (Danner et al. 2016; Fairburn et al. 2009; Harrison et al. 2010; Treasure and Schmidt 2013; Wildes et al. 2014). Being severely underweight can further compromise a person's ability to recognize and process emotions. Calls for explicit measurement of emotional and valuational factors in mental capacity assessments have been made by some authors (Hermann et al. 2016; Kious 2015). More research is needed to shed light on these issues. Hope et al. (2013) outlined several other subtle ways in which AN may compromise autonomy that procedural tests of capacity may not detect. These include the loss of agency/lack of voluntariness (i.e., inability of patients to act in accordance with their expressed decision, such as eating enough to put on weight), the fact that decisions based on false beliefs or strong emotions can still be expressed in terms of preferences, and the fact that patients experience ambivalent or conflicting desires regarding treatment that fluctuate over time.

Summary

It should be clear that many issues are still unresolved in the assessment of mental capacity, especially in AN. However, in clinical practice, such an assessment is sometimes required. This chapter attempted to provide some guidance as to how to go about this assessment. Keep in mind that the assessment of mental capacity is not an exact science; to a certain degree, this process is still surrounded by uncertainties. Careful assessment can minimize them, but clinicians should still be able to deal with uncertainty up to some point.

Clues that mental capacity may be diminished can be found in clinical variables. A low BMI, previous treatment for AN, and little appreciation of the nature and severity of the illness and the need for treatment are indications that one should be alert for diminished mental capacity. During the assessment, spend time on patients' values regarding life and death and on the meaning of AN in their life. Caretakers can be important in this part of the assessment. Evaluators should be aware that their own values may differ markedly from those of the patient and that personal values influence the decision making of the patient regarding treatment. Furthermore, any decision by the patient regarding treatment has meaning in that patient's relationships to others. Autonomy does not equal deciding in a relational vacuum. Especially in complex cases, using the MacCAT-T alongside clinical judgment can improve the assessment of mental capacity. In this way, clinicians must consciously check areas of mental capacity that might be taken for granted. Combining the clinical assessment with an eye for values, interpersonal issues, and appreciation of illness, as well as the more quantitative assessment by the MacCAT-T, can help the clinician profit from the merits of both ways of assessing mental capacity. In this manner, the mental capacity assessment is done thoroughly and with attention to the unique personal circumstances of the patient.

When clinicians judge patients to have insufficient mental capacity to refuse treatment, this does not mean the patients should no longer have any say in treatment. Even in this situation, physicians should strive to treat patients with respect for their wishes. Issues of control will remain important for patients with AN, and any area in which they can decide together with the treatment team (e.g., timing of the coerced treatment, how to go about it, when to stop with the compulsory treatment) is an opportunity to show that control has not wholly been taken from them and that they are still being taken seriously.

Conclusion

More research into assessing mental capacity in patients with AN is clearly needed. Translational cooperation between clinicians and biomedical researchers will benefit this necessary research. Quantitative studies can shed more light on the proportion of mental capacity problems in AN. To date, only one such study has been done in adults and two small studies in adolescents (Elzakkers et al. 2016; Tan et al. 2003b; Turrell et al. 2011). Replication studies are needed, and replication in populations of involuntarily treated patients can inform clinicians as to whether the proportion of mental capacity problems is even higher in this group. It would be clinically very relevant to have more information on this matter.

More exploration into what underlies mental capacity problems in patients with EDs is needed. A possible future focus could be the interplay between the emotional dysregulation often found in AN and the diminished appreciation of illness and treatment. In other populations, it has been suggested that emotion dysregulation (and not emotions as such) might impact decision making (Ayre et al. 2017; Heilman et al. 2010). In future studies, the interrater reliability of clinical judgment regarding capacity should be determined by asking two different clinicians to judge the mental capacity of the same patient, because this has not yet been studied in patients with AN. In other populations, interrater reliability regarding the mental capacity assessment between clinicians is low. In these studies, a comparison of clinical judgment and MacCAT-T could be incorporated, as well as a design in which the MacCAT-T is used in combination with clinical judgment to see whether clinical judgment is changed by use of this instrument. The issue of which assessment method is more valid is as yet unresolved. If studies reveal high interrater reliability between clinicians, then the question remains as to which assessment is more valid. If reliability proves low, this would scientifically speak in favor of a larger role for the MacCAT-T in the assessment of capacity in AN. Qualitative studies are suggested, in particular to study what issues in the clinical picture of patients with AN drive clinical judgment toward mental capacity problems.

In the field of legal-ethical studies, future studies in patients and their relatives could inform the ongoing discussion about the presumed dominance of autonomy in mental capacity assessments and how to incorporate care ethics into clinical practice. This discussion touches on the concept of mental capacity and could potentially influence the way mental capacity is assessed in clinical practice.

References

American Psychiatric Association: Diagnostic and Statistical Manual of Mental Disorders, 5th Edition. Arlington, VA, American Psychiatric Association, 2013

Applebaum PS, Grisso T: Assessing patient's capacities to consent to treatment. N Engl J Med 319(25):1635–1638, 1988

Appelbaum PS, Roth LH: Competency to consent to research: a psychiatric overview. Arch Gen Psychiatry 39(8):951–958, 1982

Ayre K, Owen GS, Moran P: Mental capacity and borderline personality disorder. B J Psychiatry Bull 41(1):43–46, 2017

Baker JH, Schaumberg K, Munn-Chernoff MA: Genetics of anorexia nervosa. Curr Psychiatry Rep 19:84, 2017

Beauchamp TL, Childress JF: Principles of Biomedical Ethics. New York, Oxford University Press, 1979

Benau EM, Orloffa NC, Janke EA, et al: A systemic review of the effects of experimental fasting on cognition. Appetite 77:52–61, 2014

Breden TM, Vollmann J: The cognitive based approach of capacity assessment in psychiatry: a philosophical critique of the MacCAT-T. Health Care Anal 12(4):273–283, discussion 265–272, 2004

Bruch H: The Golden Cage. Cambridge, MA, Harvard University Press, 1978

Buchanan AE, Brock DW: Deciding for others: The ethics of surrogate decision making. Cambridge, UK, Cambridge University Press, 1989

Cairns R, Maddock C, Buchanan A, et al: Reliability of mental capacity assessments in psychiatric in-patients. Br J Psychiatry 187:372–378, 2005

Cale GS: Risk-related standards of competence: continuing the debate over risk-related standards of competence. Bioethics 13(2):131–148, 1999

Calugi S, Chignola E, El Ghoch M, Dalle Grave R: Starvation symptoms in patients with anorexia nervosa: a longitudinal study. Eat Disord 26(6):523–537, 2018

Candia PC, Barba AC: Mental capacity and consent to treatment in psychiatric patients: the state of the research. Curr Opin Psychiatry 24(5):442–446, 2011

Carpenter WT, Gold JM, Lahti AC: Decisional capacity for informed consent in schizophrenia research. Arch Gen Psychiatry 57(6):533–538, 2000

Cavedini P, Zorci C, Bassi, T et al: Decision-making functioning as a predictor of treatment outcome in anorexia nervosa. Psychiatry Res 145(2–3):179–187, 2006

Charland LC: Appreciation and emotion: theoretical reflections on the MacArthur Treatment Competence Study. Kennedy Instit Ethics J 8(4):359–376, 1998

Charland LC: Anorexia and the MacCAT-T test for mental competence, validity, value, and emotion. Philos Psychiatry Psychol 13(4):283–287, 2007

Charland LC: Decision-making capacity, in The Stanford Encyclopedia of Philosophy, Fall 2015 Edition. Edited by Zalta EN. Stanford, CA, Stanford University, 2015

Damasio AR: Descartes' error and the future of human life. Sci Am 271(4):144, 1994

Damasio AR: The somatic marker hypothesis and the possible functions of the prefrontal cortex. Phil Trans R Soc Lon B Biol Sci 351(1346):1413–1420, 1996

Danner UN, Sternheim L, Bijsterbosch JM, et al: Influence of negative affect on decision making in women with restrictive and binge-purge type anorexia nervosa. Psychiatry Res 239:39–46, 2016

Decker JH, Fignr B, Steinglass JE: On weight and waiting: delay discounting in anorexia nervosa pretreatment and posttreatment. Biol Psychiatry 78(9):606–614, 2015

DeMarco JP: Competence and paternalism. Bioethics 16(3):231–245, 2002

den Hartogh G: Do we need a threshold conception of competence? Med Health Care Philos 19:71–83, 2016

Elzakkers IFFM, Danner UN, Hoek HW, van Elburg AA: Mental capacity to consent to treatment in anorexia nervosa: explorative study. BJPsych Open 2(2):147–153, 2016

Elzakkers IFFM, Danner UN, Sternheim LC, et al: Mental capacity to consent to treatment and the association with outcome: a longitudinal study in patients with anorexia nervosa. BJPsych Open 3(3):147–153, 2017

Elzakkers IFFM, Danner UN, Grisso T, et al: Assessment of mental capacity to consent to treatment in anorexia nervosa: a comparison of clinical judgment and MacCAT-T and consequences for clinical practice. Int J Law Psychiatry 58:27–35, 2018

Fairburn CG, Shafran R, Cooper Z: A cognitive behavioural theory of anorexia nervosa. Behav Res Ther 37(1):1–13, 1999

Fairburn CG, Cooper Z, Doll HA, et al: Transdiagnostic cognitive-behavioral therapy for patients with eating disorders: a two-site trial with 60-week follow-up. Am J Psychiatry 166(3):311–319, 2009

Fernandez-Aranda F, Pinheiro AP, Tozzi F, et al: Symptom profile of major depressive disorder in women with eating disorders Aust NZ J Psychiatry 41(1):24–31, 2007

Fladung AK, Grön G, Grammar K, et al: A neural signature of anorexia nervosa in the ventral striatal reward system. Am J Psychiatry 167(2):206–212, 2010

Foerde K, Steinglass J, Shohamy D, Walsh BT: Neural mechanisms supporting maladaptive food choices in anorexia nervosa. Nat Neurosci 18(11):1571–1573, 2015

Freedman B: Competence: marginal and otherwise. Int J Law Psychiatry 4(1–2):53–72, 1981

Grisso T, Appelbaum PS: Appreciating anorexia: decisional capacity and the role of values. Philos Psychiatry Psychol 13(4):293–301, 2006

Grisso T, Appelbaum PS, Hill-Fotouhi C: The MacCAT-T: a clinical tool to assess patients' capacities to make treatment decisions. Psychiatr Serv 48(11):1415–1419, 1997

Harrison A, Sullivan S, Tchanturia K, Treasure J: Emotional functioning in eating disorders: attentional bias, emotion recognition and emotion regulation. Psychol Med 40(11):1887–1897, 2010

Hay PJ, Sachdev P: Brain dysfunction in anorexia nervosa: cause or consequence of under-nutrition? Curr Opin Psychiatry 24(3):251–256, 2011

Heilman RM, Crisan LG, Houser D, et al: Emotion regulation and decision making under risk and uncertainty. Emotion 10:257–265, 2010

Hermann H, Trachsel M, Elger BS, Biller-Andorno N: Emotion and value in the evaluation of medical decision-making capacity: a narrative review of arguments. Front Psychol 7:765, 2016

Hindmarch T, Hotopf M, Owen G: Depression and decision-making capacity for treatment or research: a systematic review. BMC Med Ethics14(1):54, 2013

Hoek HW: Incidence, prevalence and mortality of anorexia nervosa and other eating disorders. Curr Opin Psychiatry 19(4):389–394, 2006

Hope H, Tan J, McMillian J: Agency, ambivalence and authenticity: the many ways in which anorexia nervosa can affect autonomy. Int J Law Context 9(1):20–36, 2013

Hotopf M: The assessment of mental capacity. Clin Med (Lond) 5(6):580–584, 2005

Kaye WH, Wierenga CE, Bailer UF, et al: Nothing tastes as good as skinny feels: the neurobiology of anorexia nervosa. Trends Neurosci 36(2):110–120, 2013

Keating C: Theoretical perspective on anorexia nervosa: the conflict of reward. Neurosci Biobehav Rev 34(1):73–79, 2010

Keski-Rahkonen A, Hoek HW, Susser ES, et al: Epidemiology and course of anorexia nervosa in the community. Am J Psychiatry 164(8):1259–1265, 2007

Keys A, Brožek J, Henschel A, et al: The Biology of Human Starvation. St. Paul, MN, University of Minnesota Press, 1950

Kious BM: Autonomy and values: why the conventional theory of autonomy is not value-neutral. Philos Psychiatry Psychol 22(1):1–12, 2015

Kitamura T, Kitamura F: Reliability of clinical judgment of patients' competency to give informed consent: a case vignette study. Psychiatry Clin Neurosci 54(2):245–247, 2000

Lao-Kaim NP, Fonville L, Giampietro VP, et al: Aberrant function of learning and cognitive control networks underlie inefficient cognitive flexibility in anorexia nervosa: a cross-sectional fMRI study. PLoS ONE 10(5), 2015

Lapid MI, Rummans TA, Poole KL, et al: Decisional capacity of severely depressed patients requiring electroconvulsive therapy. J ECT 19(2):67–72, 2003

Lapid MI, Rummans TA, Pankratz VS, Appelbaum PS: Decisional capacity of depressed elderly to consent to electroconvulsive therapy. J Geriatr Psychiatry Neurol 17(1):42–46, 2004

Lepping P: Overestimating patients' capacity. Br J Psychiatry 199(5):355–356, 2011

Lepping P, Sambhi RS, Williams-Jones K: Deprivation of liberty safeguards: how prepared are we? J Med Ethics 36(3):170–173, 2010

Marson DC, McInturff B, Hawkins L: Consistency of physician judgments of capacity to consent in mild Alzheimer's disease. J Am Geriatr Soc 45(4):453–457, 1997

Naqvi N, Shiv B, Bechara A: The role of emotion in decision making: a cognitive neuroscience perspective. Cur Dir Psychol Sci 15(5):260–264, 2006

Okai D, Owen G, McGuire H, et al: Mental capacity in psychiatric patients: systematic review. Br J Psychiatry 191:291–297, 2007

Owen GS, Szmukler G, Richardson G, et al: Decision-making capacity for treatment in psychiatric and medical in-patients: cross-sectional, comparative study. Br J Psychiatry 203(6):461–467, 2013

Phillipou A, Rossell SL, Castle DJ: The neurobiology of anorexia nervosa: a systematic review. Aust NZ J Psychiatry 48(2):128–152, 2014

Phillipou A, Rossell SL, Castle DJ: Anorexia nervosa or starvation? Eur J Neurosci 48(11):3317–3318, 2018

Piech RM, Hampshire A, Owen AM, Parkinson JA: Modulation of cognitive flexibility by hunger and desire. Cogn Emot 23(3):528–540, 2009

Polivy J: Psychological consequences of food restriction. J Am Diet Assoc 96(6):589–592, 1996

Raney TJ, Thornton LM, Berrettini W, et al: Influence of overanxious disorder of childhood on the expression of anorexia nervosa. Int J Eat Disord 41(4):326–332, 2008

Remmers C, Michalak J: Losing your gut feelings: intuition in depression. Front Psychol 7:1291, 2016

Roth LH, Meisel A, Lidz CW: Tests of competency to consent to treatment. Am J Psychiatry 134(3):279–284, 1977

Shafran R, de Silva P: Cognitive-behavioural models, in Handbook of Eating Disorders. Hoboken, NJ, John Wiley and Sons, 2005, pp 121–138

Shah A, Mukherjee S: Ascertaining capacity to consent: a survey of approaches used by psychiatrists. Med Sci Law 43(3):231–235, 2003

Smink FR, van Hoeken D, Hoek HW: Epidemiology of eating disorders: incidence, prevalence and mortality rates. Curr Psychiatry Rep 14(4):406–414, 2012

Steinhausen HC: The outcome of anorexia nervosa in the 20th century. Am J Psychiatry 159(8):1284–1293, 2002

Støving RK: Anorexia nervosa and endocrinology: a clinical update. Eur J Endocrinol 180(1):R9–R27, 2019

Sturman ED: The capacity to consent to treatment and research: a review of standardized assessment tools. Clin Psychol Rev 25(7):954–974, 2005

Tan J: The anorexia talking? Lancet 362(3):1246–1246, 2003

Tan J, McMillan JR: The discrepancy between the legal definition of capacity and the British Medical Association's guidelines. J Med Ethics 30(5):427–429, 2004

Tan J, Hope T, Stewart A: Anorexia and personal identity: the accounts of patients and their parents. Int J Law Psychiatry 26(5):533–548, 2003a

Tan J, Hope T, Stewart A: Competence to refuse treatment in anorexia nervosa. Int J Law Psychiatry 26(6):697–707, 2003b

Tan J, Hope T, Stewart A, Fitzpatrick R: Control and compulsory treatment in anorexia nervosa: the views of patients and parents Int J Law Psychiatry 26(6):267–245, 2003c

Tan J, Stewart A, Fitzpatrick R, Hope T: Studying penguins to understand birds. Philos Psychiatry Psychol 13(4):299–301, 2006

Tan J, Stewart A, Hope T: Decision-making as a broader concept. Philos Psychiatry Psychol 16(4):345–349, 2009

Tchanturia K, Morris RG, Brecelj M, et al: Set shifting in anorexia nervosa: an examination before and after weight gain, in full recovery and relationship to childhood and adult OCPD traits. J Psychiatr Res 38(5):545–552, 2004

Tchanturia K, Liao PC, Uher R, et al: An investigation of decision making in anorexia nervosa using the Iowa Gambling Task and skin conductance measurements. J Int Neuropsychol Soc 13(4):635–641, 2007

Treasure J, Schmidt U: The cognitive-interpersonal maintenance model of anorexia nervosa revisited: a summary of the evidence for cognitive, socio-emotional and interpersonal predisposing and perpetuating factors. J Eat Disord 1:13, 2013

Turrell SL, Peterson-Badali M, Katzman DK: Consent to treatment in adolescents with anorexia nervosa. Int J Eat Disord 44(8):703–707, 2011

Vellinga A, Smit JH, Van Leeuwen E, et al: Competence to consent to treatment of geriatric patients: judgements of physicians, family members and the vignette method. Int J Geriatr Psychiatry 19(7):645–654, 2004

Vollmann J: "But I don't feel it": values and emotions in the assessment of competence in patients with anorexia nervosa. Philos Psychiatry, Psychol 13(4):289–291, 2006

Vollmann J, Bauer A, Danker-Hopfe H, Helmchen H: Competence of mentally ill patients: a comparative empirical study. Psychol Med 33(8):1463–1471, 2003

Wang SB, Wang YY, Ungvari GS, et al: The MacArthur Competence Assessment Tools for assessing decision-making capacity in schizophrenia: a meta-analysis. Schizophr Res 183:56–63, 2017

Wildes JE, Marcus MD, Cheng Y, et al: Emotion acceptance behavior therapy for anorexia nervosa: a pilot study. Int J Eat Disord 47(8):870–873, 2014

Wu M, Brockmeyer T, Hartmann M, et al: Reward-related decision making in eating and weight disorders: a systematic review and meta-analysis of the evidence from neuropsychological studies. Neurosci Biobehav Rev 61:177–196, 2016

Zink CF, Weinberger DR: Cracking the moody brain: the reward of self starvation. Nat Med 16(12):1382–1383, 2010

5

Role of Medical Guardianship

Dennis Gibson, M.D.
Philip S. Mehler, M.D.
Patricia Westmoreland, M.D.

THE ethical and legal issues surrounding compulsory treatment of individuals with eating disorders (EDs) are made even more challenging given the high mortality rate of these disorders and the difficulty in treating them effectively. Indeed, after only opioid abuse, anorexia nervosa (AN) has the highest mortality of all mental health illnesses, with a standardized mortality ratio of nearly 6% per decade, related to both medical complications from the malnutrition and increased rates of suicide (Chesney et al. 2014). Given the ego-syntonic nature of this disease, patients are often unaware of the severity of their malnutrition, their risk for poor medical outcomes, or even that they have an ED. Therefore, they are frequently unwilling to admit the need for therapeutic intervention and often refuse treatment when offered. Medical guardianship grants legal authority to make medical decisions for another person who is thought to be incapable of making such decisions regarding his or her own health.

In this chapter, we outline the medical complications that can develop from extreme malnutrition. We then discuss the role of guardianship in caring for people with severe EDs. Finally, we discuss how guardianship in the United States differs from guardianship laws in other parts of the world.

Medical Consequences of Severe Eating Disorders

EDs are all-encompassing, multisystem diseases that contribute to the development of medical complications in every organ system. These complications are a function of both the extent of starvation and the method of purging.

Dermatological changes in people with malnutrition include xerosis (dry skin), lanugo (hypertrichosis lanuginosa), telogen effluvium, increased nail fragility, and acrocyanosis (Strumia 2013). These are expected physiological manifestations of starvation, with possible contribution from micronutrient deficiencies. Lanugo presents as fine downy hair that largely serves to conserve heat. Telogen effluvium is diffuse, reversible hair loss caused by an increasing number of hair follicles entering the resting phase of growth. Acrocyanosis occurs due to abnormal functioning of blood vessels that likely serves as an energy-conserving mechanism. These changes are all reversible with weight restoration. People engaging in self-induced vomiting can also develop a pathognomonic finding called Russell's sign, which is thickening of the skin over the dorsal surface of the knuckles.

Changes of the head, ears, eyes, nose, and throat include lagophthalmos (an inability to fully close the eyelids), which can cause eye irritation (Gaudiani et al. 2012), autophonia (hyperperception of one's voice) (Godbole and Key 2010), and oropharyngeal dysphagia due to weakness of the swallowing muscles (Holmes et al. 2016). Lagophthalmos and autophonia likely develop due to loss of fatty tissue surrounding the orbit and Eustachian tube, respectively. These conditions are fully reversible with weight restoration. Complications prone to develop in those engaging in self-induced vomiting can include an increased risk of dental caries (Strumia 2013); perimylolysis (erosion of the lingual surface of the teeth) (Strumia 2013); subconjunctival hemorrhage and epistaxis due to forced retching; and sialadenosis, or hypertrophy of the salivary glands, most notably the parotid glands (Vavrina et al. 1994).

Cardiac manifestations of malnutrition include generalized atrophy, mitral valve prolapse, and pericardial effusion. The cardiac atrophy and dimensional changes that develop due to malnutrition contribute to laxity of the mitral valve as seen in mitral valve prolapse (Meyers et al. 1987). Pericardial effusion, or fluid in the sac surrounding the heart, develops in a sizable number of patients for unclear reasons and rarely causes any symptoms unless a significant amount of fluid develops, leading to cardiac tamponade (Kastner et al. 2012). Sinus bradycardia and other bradyarrhythmias occur with greater frequency in these patients, likely due to increased vagal tone

(Petretta et al. 1997; Yahalom et al. 2013). Hypotension is also a common finding, for similar reasons. Sudden cardiac death, which can likely be attributed to structural cardiac changes, including significant atrophy and cardiac scarring as well as increased QT dispersion (differences in the QT measurement between each lead on the electrocardiogram), all predispose to increased risk for arrhythmias and mortality in this population (Krantz et al. 2005; Lamzabi et al. 2015). High-risk arrhythmias are also more likely to occur in those who purge, as a result of the secondary electrolyte deficiencies that develop (Crow et al. 2009). These findings are reversible with weight restoration.

Pulmonary complications are a less common manifestation of starvation but, nonetheless, are an important consideration in people with severe EDs. Complications may include spontaneous pneumothorax and pneumomediastinum (Jensen et al. 2017; Lee et al. 2015). These changes seem to develop secondary to nontraumatic alveolar rupture and thus are no more common in those who purge than in those who solely restrict their caloric intake. Aspiration pneumonia may also develop in those who engage in purging via vomiting.

Gastrointestinal complaints are the most frequently reported symptoms in patients with ED (Norris et al. 2016), due not only to changes in physiological functioning of the gastrointestinal tract but also to the high prevalence of functional disease in this population. Gastroparesis, manifesting as abdominal fullness, nausea, and bloating, is a nearly universal finding in people with significant malnutrition. Patients also frequently complain of constipation. Gastroparesis and slow-transit constipation are likely physiological adaptations of malnutrition, allowing for the optimal uptake of nutrients as food travels through the gastrointestinal tract. Patients also often complain of loose stools as they start refeeding because of intestinal villous atrophy that develops secondary to the malnutrition, a finding supported by reduced serum diamine oxidase (Takimoto et al. 2014). Individuals with malnutrition secondary to EDs also seem to be at risk for pancreatic injury and rectal prolapse (Norris et al. 2016). With the possible exception of rectal prolapse, these conditions are expected to normalize with weight restoration.

Superior mesenteric artery (SMA) syndrome is another potential gastrointestinal complication of malnutrition that can develop in patients with EDs (Mascolo et al. 2015; Norris et al. 2016). The SMA, which branches off the aorta, can undergo medial migration with loss of the fat pad that supports it. This migration causes the second part of the duodenum to become compressed between the SMA and the aorta. Patients complain of abdominal pain that occurs after consuming meals and is relieved with emesis or the passage of time from meal completion. Surgery is not recommended for this condition because weight restoration alone will build up the fat pad and allow the SMA to migrate back into the appropriate position, thereby releasing compression of the duodenum and allowing easier passage of the chyme. Gastric dilatation is a rare complication that can also develop in those with SMA syndrome or some other downstream obstruction (Mascolo et al. 2015); this should be treated as an emergency given the propensity for gastric perforation to develop.

People who engage in purging are at further risk for gastrointestinal complications depending on their mode of purging. Those who purge via emesis are at increased risk for gastroesophageal reflux disease not only as a result of the gastroparesis, which increases risk for backup of stomach contents into the esophagus, but also due to the gastric acid that contacts the esophageal tissue during emesis (Norris et al. 2016). Furthermore, ongoing emesis will eventually damage the lower esophageal sphincter, increasing the likelihood of stomach contents entering the esophagus. Forced retching can also increase the risk for hematemesis via Mallory-Weiss tears as well as, rarely, esophageal rupture. Those who abuse stimulant laxatives may be at risk for cathartic colon (Smith 1972), a condition whereby the large intestine becomes an inert tube incapable of peristalsis, thus predisposing to constipation. This condition frequently resolves with discontinuation of the stimulant laxatives.

Malnutrition has direct effects on the liver as well, increasing the risk for starvation hepatitis (Rosen et al. 2017). Starvation hepatitis is increasingly common as the extent of malnutrition worsens. The hepatocytes undergo autophagy (apoptosis) as a means to increase nutrients for the rest of the body. The abnormally elevated alanine aminotransferase and aspartate aminotransferase seen in this condition will normalize with weight restoration; however, ongoing monitoring of liver function tests is required with nutritional rehabilitation due to the additional risk of refeeding hepatitis, an inflammatory condition of the liver that can develop during refeeding.

Individuals with malnutrition often present with leukopenia (low white blood cells) and normocytic anemia and less often with thrombocytopenia (low platelets) (Sabel et al. 2013). Often, the bone marrow is replaced by a gelatinous extracellular matrix rich in hyaluronic acid, leading to a condition known as gelatinous marrow transformation (Sabel et al. 2013). These cell counts will normalize with weight restoration. Even with the frequent leukopenia and neutropenia, these individuals do not appear to be at increased risk for infection.

Worsening malnutrition leads to weakness and deconditioning as a result of increased muscle atrophy (McLoughlin et al. 1998). Gray- and white-matter neurological changes also develop secondary to worsening malnutrition (Seitz et al. 2016). Although muscle atrophy and gray matter changes seem to normalize with weight restoration, it is unclear whether the white matter deficiencies that are manifested as abnormalities in multiple neural pathways fully normalize with weight restoration or if these white matter deficiencies are actually a trait-dependent finding that ultimately contributes to the development of the eating disorder (Bosanac et al. 2007).

Deficits in multiple hormonal axes can develop secondary to malnutrition (Miller 2011). The hypothalamic-pituitary-adrenal axis becomes dysregulated resulting in increased cortisol. This can have secondary effects on the body, including increased risk of osteoporosis and gastritis and upregulation of gluconeogenesis, which acts to combat the hypoglycemia these patients tend to develop. The hypothalamic-pituitary-thyroid axis also becomes dysregulated, with frequently low to low-normal levels of free thyroxine and thyroid-stimulating hormone, low triiodothyronine (T3), and increased reverse T3, thus appearing similar to sick euthyroid syndrome. Functioning of the hypothalamic-pituitary-gonadal axis also slows in patients with EDs, manifesting with low sex hormones, which leads to amenorrhea in females and testosterone deficiency in males. Other hormonal changes include leptin deficiency and growth hormone resistance, manifesting as low insulin-like growth factor.

As the extent of malnutrition increases, hypoglycemia becomes more common due to lack of glycogen stores from prolonged fasting as well as lack of substrate for gluconeogenesis (Mehler and Andersen 2017). Hypoglycemia is a likely risk for sudden death, and these patients often manifest with hypoglycemic unawareness, suggesting that their bodies have adapted to recurrent hypoglycemia and the usual autonomic and neurohormonal changes that occur with hypoglycemia no longer develop.

Bone disease is another medical complication noted to develop in individuals with severe malnutrition (Drabkin et al. 2017). Multiple factors increase the risk for developing low bone density, such as increased cortisol, growth hormone resistance, sex hormone deficiency, more exercise when at a low body weight, decreased leptin, and abnormal levels of appetite-regulating hormones that also regulate bone structure. Weight restoration ultimately improves bone density, with or without use of pharmacological agents, although bone density may not improve to a normal level.

Refeeding syndrome is one of the most feared consequences of treating patients with EDs. Full-blown refeeding syndrome is characterized by cardiac failure, hemolysis, rhabdomyolysis, seizures, and electrolyte deficiencies of phosphorous and potassium; severe cases of refeeding syndrome can result in death. Hypophosphatemia alone is often noted as patients start to refeed and becomes more common at lower body weights (Brown et al. 2015). This syndrome can be prevented with close monitoring and correction of hypophosphatemia. Hypokalemia can also develop outside refeeding syndrome in those who use various methods of purging; pure calorie restrictors rarely develop hypokalemia strictly due to lack of appropriate food intake. Recurrent hypokalemia can contribute to the development of hypokalemic nephropathy, which can lead to chronic kidney disease (Chih-Chia and Hung-Chieh 2011). Hyponatremia can also develop in patients with EDs, secondary either to deficient or excessive fluid intake (primary polydipsia) (Bahia et al. 2011). Hypernatremia is occasionally noted, with central diabetes insipidus potentially contributing (Rosen et al. 2019).

Pseudo-Bartter syndrome is another potential complication for patients who purge, regardless of the extent of malnutrition (Bahia et al. 2012). Ongoing frequent purging leads to intravascular depletion, which contributes to upregulation of the renin-angiotensin-aldosterone axis. Aldosterone acts to increase sodium reabsorption in the renal tubules, with secondary water absorption, predisposing to the development of edema and excessive weight gain. Treatment requires cessation of purging; the aldosterone antagonist spironolactone can be used until aldosterone levels have normalized, which usually takes about 2–3 weeks after purging stops.

As should now be clear, the medical complications of EDs affect almost every organ system and become increasingly severe with greater extent of malnutrition. These physical manifestations are largely reversible, with the possible exception of low bone mineral density for age and neurological white matter deficits. However, patients frequently refuse the treatment (i.e., nutrition) needed to remedy these complications, some of which require specialized treatment on a medical unit before a severely ill person is medically stable enough to be admitted to an inpatient ED treatment unit. Guardianship is a method whereby families may pursue medical treatment for a family member who is refusing treatment of a severe eating disorder.

Role of Guardianship

Medical guardianship is one legal tool that allows for substituted decision making for individuals with EDs. Lack of a perceived need for treatment is a common barrier to medical intervention for people with mental illness (Mojtabai et al. 2011), and those with EDs are especially prone to a lack of insight into the nature and gravity of their illness, especially given the ego-syntonic nature of most EDs (Gregertsen et al. 2017).

A *guardian* is someone tasked with exercising substituted judgment on behalf of a person determined to be incapacitated (i.e., the ward) (National Guardianship Association 2019). The process of obtaining guardianship first requires a capacity evaluation—that is, a determination of whether the person in question can make an informed decision regarding a specific task.

Capacity is defined as individuals' ability to understand information about their condition, appreciate the consequences of the decisions they make, capably reason through the information needed to make these decisions, and then communicate their choices (Appelbaum and Grisso 1988). With regard to EDs, capacity ultimately revolves around the person's ability to understand that he or she has an ED; the nature, severity, and consequences of that ED; and that adequate nutritional intake and cessation of purging (if relevant) are required to successfully treat that ED and prevent further morbidity and mortality. If the person is deemed to lack capacity, which is a medical opinion, the case is presented to the court to determine whether the person is *competent*, which is a legal finding. If the person is deemed incompetent, guardianship can be granted at the court's discretion.

However, the role of the medical guardian as it relates to treatment in AN, which is considered a mental health illness, is limited. Guardians are capable of making decisions about a ward's medical care but not for the psychiatric component of the illness (Westmoreland et al. 2017). Guardianship does not grant a guardian the power to admit a ward to a mental health facility without the ward's consent. Furthermore, once a ward is no longer medically compromised, ongoing psychiatric care and nutritional rehabilitation can only be authorized by the courts under the guise of civil commitment (Westmoreland et al. 2017).

Treatment of EDs is inherently paternalistic, given the ego-syntonic nature of the disease. Guardianship may further increase the amount of perceived coercion experienced by the patient during treatment (Matusek and Wright 2010). Kendall (2014) argued that coercion is a justifiable component of treatment because patients with EDs often inherently do not have competence; their identities are "enmeshed in the pathology of their illness" and autonomy is lost if their personal identity is altered by the disease. However, this single argument does not resolve the ethical dilemma of paternalism versus patient autonomy as it relates to patients with EDs, and in some cases, even though patients may not have decision-making capacity regarding treatment for their ED, they are still thought to have the capacity to judge the extent of their own suffering and quality of life, especially if the latter has not been improved by multiple rounds of treatment (Lopez et al. 2010; Yager 2015).

The role of the guardian in the treatment of patients with EDs also presents legal dilemmas. The legal definition of being medically compromised and needing emergent therapeutic intervention is not well defined with respect to medical complications that develop in these patients. Obviously, one can easily justify the need for urgent medical intervention when the patient presents with, for example, hypoglycemia, electrolyte abnormalities, and some heart arrhythmias, which are clearly associated with increased mortality. Although a greater degree of malnutrition predisposes to an increased likelihood of medical complications, one can still not predict when these complications will develop or even at what weight a particular individual might experience sudden death. Furthermore, if nutritional intervention is started against a patient's will, at what percent ideal body weight will the ward no longer be considered medically compromised and hence capable of refusing additional nutrition under guardianship regulations?

Similarly, no legal decisions have been made regarding the need for intervention in patients who develop medical complications that could ultimately increase their risk for sudden death. For example, starvation hepatitis, a complication in which the liver undergoes cell death to provide nutrients for the rest of the body, is associated with development of hypoglycemia (Rosen et al. 2017). Therefore, should a guardian be able to override patient autonomy when a complication arises that predisposes to a secondary condition associated with increased mortality, even if that secondary condition has not yet developed? Malnutrition places severe stress on various body systems. Does it follow, then, that any medical complication arising from the malnutrition constitutes a situation in which emergent medical intervention is justified, even against the patient's wishes, given that the severity of malnutrition is not expected to improve without intervention?

These questions are currently difficult to answer, given the paucity of research regarding the use of guardianship for the treatment of those with EDs. Griffiths et al. (1997) performed a small retrospective study examining the use of guardianship for treatment of AN. Results indicated slower rates of weight gain, increased morbidity, and increased numbers of prior treatments for those treated under guardianship. All of the subjects who were treated under guardianship initially denied their illness and refused treatment, which further supported the use of guardianship in these situations. These patients eventually acquired similar BMIs at time of discharge to those not treated under guardianship. However, follow-up was inadequate to draw conclusions as to guardianship's effects on treatment. Furthermore, this study was conducted in New South Wales, Australia, which allows compulsory treatment under guardianship, so findings should not be extrapolated to potential outcomes in the United States. Similarly, Born et al. (2015) examined outcomes of severely ill individuals with AN at a psychiatric inpatient unit that required legal guardianship be in place for admittance. The study was conducted in Germany, where guardianship allows for compulsory care, so findings again cannot be extrapolated to possible outcomes in the United States. No studies have examined the frequency of guardianship use in the United States or the outcomes of patients treated under guardianship under current U.S. laws. Finally, no research has examined the use of nutritional intervention for those with EDs under guardianship in this country.

Guardianship in the United States

Because the definition of *incapacity*, and therefore ultimately *guardianship*, is determined by the state, more than 50 guardianship systems exist in the United States. The Uniform Adult Guardianship and Protective Proceedings Jurisdiction Act (UAGPPJA; National Conference of Commissioners on Uniform State Laws 2007) was established to help navigate the legal requirements of guardianship by state. It allows transfer of guardianship between states with the goal of minimizing, or even eliminating, the need for additional legal proceedings. The guardian must petition the court in the state currently holding the guardianship and request to move the application to another state. This relocation must be in the ward's best interests; the plans for the ward's care must be "reasonable and sufficient"; objections, if any, to the relocation must have been addressed; and the relocation must be permanent. However, as of this writing, the UAGPPJA has still not been adopted in all 50 states, with Florida, Kansas, Michigan, Texas, and Wisconsin not having passed legislation to this effect.

Guardianship in Other Countries

Mental health laws and the role of the guardian in the treatment of mental health differ around the world. For example, in New South Wales, Australia, patients with EDs can receive compulsory treatment through two separate laws. One, the Mental Health Act 2007 (Department of Health 2007) defines *mental illness* as

> a condition that seriously impairs, either temporarily or permanently, the mental functioning of a person and is characterized by the presence in the person of any one of the following symptoms: a) delusions, b) hallucinations, c) serious disorder of thought form, d) a severe disturbance of mood, and/or e) sustained or repeated irrational behavior indicating the presence of any one or more of the symptoms.

A person must also be at risk of serious harm, and involuntary care must be the least restrictive form of care, for that person to receive compulsory care under this Act. It allows mandated treatment in declared mental health facilities or medical wards and includes nutritional restoration (Johnson et al. 2017). However, it does not allow for involuntary treatment at nondesignated facilities or private ED clinics.

The second law, the Guardianship Act 1987 (2014), also allows for compulsory treatment of those with EDs. It allows for the same compulsory care and forms of intervention as the Mental Health Act 2007, but treatment is pursued under the definition of *disability*: "a person who is restricted in one or more major life activities to such an extent that he or she requires supervision," of which an ED can be classified. This restriction may be because of an intellectual, physical, or psychological disability or because the person is mentally ill. The Guardianship Act 1987 allows for treatment at facilities besides those allowed by the Mental Health Act 2007, including nondeclared medical wards or public hospitals as well as private ED clinics (Johnson et al. 2017), thereby allowing for continued involuntary care after discharge from an inpatient facility. The order also allows for a longer duration of nutritional intervention, as discussed in Griffiths et al. (1997).

Conclusion

Treatment of patients with AN and other EDs is fraught with both ethical and legal dilemmas. Given the ego-syntonic nature of EDs, patient resistance to treatment is frequently encountered, further contributing to the high mortality of these disorders. EDs can require months of weight restoration, depending on the individual's initial body weight, and greater body weight after acute treatment confers better short-term outcomes (Kaplan et al. 2009). Although guardianship may be helpful for obtaining medical treatment for a person with a serious ED, its role is limited once the medical crisis has passed. Furthermore, current mental health and guardianship jurisdiction do not allow for ongoing nutritional intervention against the will of patients with increasing body weight, thereby precluding them from receiving appropriate long-term treatment unless they enter treatment voluntarily or certification is pursued.

References

Appelbaum PS, Grisso T: Assessing patients' capacities to consent to treatment. N Engl J Med 319:1635–1638, 1988

Bahia A, Chu ES, Mehler PS: Polydipsia and hyponatremia in a woman with anorexia nervosa. Int J Eat Disord 44:186–188, 2011

Bahia A, Mascolo M, Gaudiani JL, et al: PseudoBartter syndrome in eating disorders. Int J Eat Disord 45:150–153, 2012

Born C, de la Fontaine L, Winter B, et al: First results of a refeeding program in a psychiatric intensive care unit for patients with extreme anorexia nervosa. BMC Psychiatry 15:57, 2015

Bosanac P, Kurlender S, Stojanovska L, et al: Neuropsychological study of underweight and "weight-recovered" anorexia nervosa compared with bulimia nervosa and normal controls. Int J Eat Disord 40:613–621, 2007

Brown CA, Sabel AL, Gaudiani JL, et al: Predictors of hypophosphatemia during refeeding of patients with severe anorexia nervosa. Int J Eat Disord 48:898–904, 2015

Chesney E, Goodwin GM, Fazel S: Risks of all-cause and suicide mortality in mental disorders: a meta-review. World Psychiatry 13(2):153–160, 2014

Chih-Chia L, Hung-Chieh Y: Hypokalemic nephropathy in anorexia nervosa. CMAJ 183(11):E761, 2011

Crow SJ, Peterson CB, Swanson SA, et al: Increased mortality in bulimia nervosa and other eating disorders. Am J Psychiatry 166(12):1342–1346, 2009

Department of Health: Mental Capacity Act. London, Her Majesty's Stationery Office, 2007

Drabkin A, Rothman MS, Wassenaar E, et al: Assessment and clinical management of bone disease in adults with eating disorders: a review. J Eat Disord 5:42, 2017

Gaudiani JL, Braverman JM, Mascolo M, et al: Ophthalmic changes in severe anorexia nervosa: a case series. Int J Eat Disord 45(5):719–721, 2012

Godbole M, Key A: Autophonia in anorexia nervosa. Int J Eat Disord 43:480–482, 2010

Gregertsen EC, Mandy W, Serpell L: The ego-syntonic nature of anorexia: an impediment to recovery in anorexia nervosa treatment. Front Psychol 8:2273, 2017

Griffiths RA, Beumont PJV, Russell J, et al: The use of guardianship legislation for anorexia nervosa: a report of 15 cases. Aust NZ J Psychiatry 31:525–531, 1997

Guardianship Act 1987 No 257 [NSW]. New South Wales, Australia, 2014

Holmes SRM, Sabel AL, Gaudiani JL, et al: Prevalence and management of oropharyngeal dysphagia in patients with severe anorexia nervosa: a large retrospective review. Int J Eat Disord 49(2):159–166, 2016

Jensen VM, Stoving RK, Andersen PE: Anorexia nervosa with massive pulmonary air leak and extraordinary propagation. Int J Eat Disord 50:451–453, 2017

Johnson A, Schyvens M, Maloney D: Coercive treatment options for anorexia under the mental health and guardianship acts. Law Society Journal 37:86–87, 2017

Kaplan AS, Walsh BT, Olmsted M: The slippery slope: prediction of successful weight maintenance in anorexia nervosa. Psychol Med 39(6):1037–1045, 2009

Kastner S, Salbach-Andrae H, Renneberg B, et al: Echocardiographic findings in adolescents with anorexia nervosa at beginning of treatment and after weight recovery. Eur Child Adolesc Psychiatry 21:15–21, 2012

Kendall S: Anorexia nervosa: the diagnosis. A postmodern ethics contribution to the bioethics debate on involuntary treatment for anorexia nervosa. J Bioeth Inq 11(1):31–40, 2014

Krantz MJ, Donahoo WT, Melanson EL, et al: QT interval dispersion and resting metabolic rate in chronic anorexia nervosa. Int J Eat Disord 37:166–170, 2005

Lamzabi I, Syed S, Reddy VB, et al: Myocardial changes in a patient with anorexia nervosa: a case report and review of the literature. Am J Clin Pathol 143:734–737, 2015

Lee KJ, Yun HK, Park IN: Spontaneous pneumomediastinum: an unusual pulmonary complication in anorexia nervosa. Tuberc Respir Dis (Seoul) 78:360–362, 2015

Lopez A, Yager J, Feinstein RE: Medical futility and psychiatry: palliative care and hospice care as a last resort in the treatment of refractory anorexia nervosa. Int J Eat Disord 43:372–377, 2010

Mascolo M, Dee E, Townsend R, et al: Severe gastric dilatation due to superior mesenteric artery syndrome in anorexia nervosa. Int J Eat Disord 48:532–534, 2015

Matusek JA, Wright MO: Ethical dilemmas in treating clients with eating disorders: a review and application of an integrative ethical decision-making model. Eur Eat Disord Rev 18:434–452, 2010

McLoughlin DM, Spargo E, Wassif WS, et al: Structural and functional changes in skeletal muscle in anorexia nervosa. Acta Neuropathol 95:632–640, 1998

Mehler PS, Andersen AE: Eating Disorders: A Guide to Medical Care and Complications. Baltimore, MD, John Hopkins University Press, 2017

Meyers DG, Starke H, Pearson PH, et al: Leaflet to left ventricular size disproportionate and prolapse of structurally normal mitral valve in anorexia nervosa. Am J Cardiol 60(10):911–914, 1987

Miller KK: Endocrine dysregulation in anorexia nervosa update. J Clin Endocrinol Metab 96(10):2939–2949, 2011

Mojtabai R, Olfson M, Sampson NA, et al: Barriers to mental health treatment: results from the National Comorbidity Survey Replication (NCS-R). Psychol Med 41(8):1751–1761, 2011

National Conference of Commissioners on Uniform State Laws: Uniform Adult Guardianship and Protective Proceedings Jurisdiction Act. Chicago, IL, National Conference of Commissioners on Uniform State Laws, 2007. Available at: https://www.naela.org/App_Themes/Public/PDF/Advocacy%20Tab/Uniform%20Guardianship%20Act/Final%20Act%20with%20Perfatory%20Note.pdf. Accessed August 5, 2019.

National Guardianship Association: What Is Guardianship? Bellefont, PA, National Guardianship Association, 2019. Available at: https://www.guardianship.org/what-is-guardianship. Accessed August 1 2019.

Norris ML, Harrison ME, Isserlin L, et al: Gastrointestinal complications associated with anorexia nervosa: a systematic review. Int J Eat Disord 49(3):216–237, 2016

Petretta M, Bonaduce D, Scalfi L, et al: Heart rate variability as a measure of autonomic nervous system function in anorexia nervosa. Clin Cardiol 20:219–224, 1997

Rosen E, Bakshi N, Watters A, et al: Hepatic complications of anorexia nervosa. Dig Dis Sci 62:2977–2981, 2017

Rosen E, Thambundit A, Mehler PS, et al: Central diabetes insipidus associated with refeeding in anorexia nervosa: a case report. Int J Eat Disord 52(6):752–756, 2019

Sabel AL, Gaudiani JL, Statland B, et al: Hematological abnormalities in severe anorexia nervosa. Ann Hematol 92(5):605–613, 2013

Seitz J, Herpertz-Dahlmann B, Konrad K: Brain morphological changes in adolescent and adult patients with anorexia nervosa. J Neural Trans 123(8):949–959, 2016

Smith B: Pathology of cathartic colon. Proc R Soc Med 65(3):288, 1972

Strumia R: Eating disorders and the skin. Clin Dermatol 31:80–85, 2013

Takimoto Y, Yoshiuchi K, Shimodaira S, et al: Diamine oxidase activity levels in anorexia nervosa. Int J Eat Disord 47:203–205, 2014

Vavrina J, Muller W, Gebbers JO: Enlargement of salivary glands in bulimia. J Laryngol Otol 108:516–518, 1994

Westmoreland P, Johnson C, Stafford M, et al: Involuntary treatment of patients with life-threatening anorexia nervosa. J Am Acad Psychiatry Law 45:419–425, 2017

Yager J: The futility of arguing about medical futility in anorexia nervosa: the question is how you would handle highly specific circumstances. Am J Bioethics 15:47–50, 2015

Yahalom M, Spitz M, Sandler L, et al: The significance of bradycardia in anorexia nervosa. Int J Angiol 22(2):83–94, 2013

6

Civil Commitment

Wayne Bowers, Ph.D.
Michael Stafford, J.D.
Patricia Westmoreland, M.D.

EATING disorders (EDs), especially anorexia nervosa (AN), pose physical and mental health risks, especially for those who fail to understand the seriousness of the disorder. Untreated, these disorders can become chronic conditions that interfere with a person's ability to effectively achieve normal social, psychological, academic, and occupational goals. Inherent to the ED is an inability to understand or denial of the nature or seriousness of one's condition, to the extent that treatment refusal can threaten the person's total well-being. When this occurs, civil commitment should be considered if the treating clinician believes the person no longer has the ability to assist in making decisions regarding treatment (American Psychiatric Association 2006). Civil commitment is especially warranted and clinically prudent for patients whose lives are threatened by severe EDs, and cases tried before the courts have demonstrated that courts are willing to accept the manifestations of EDs as overvalued ideas or beliefs that may require involuntary treatment (Westmoreland et al. 2017).

The evolution of modern civil commitment is a complex set of interactions among state legislatures, lay and professional interest groups, and the judicial system. Financial support from governments in the area of mental health, legislative changes at the state and federal level, and increased emphasis on personal civil rights and liberties have all shaped how and when civil commitment is used (Anfang and Appelbaum 2006; Appelbaum 2006;

Bloom 2004). People with mental illness who lack the mental capacity to assist in their own treatment, deny their illness, or refuse treatment, leading to life-threatening or -impeding outcomes, are frequently involved in civil commitment proceedings. Involuntary hospitalization has been argued as a critical first step in psychiatric care and is seen as a mainstay to initiating psychiatric care (Testa and West 2010). However, balancing the treatment needs of those with an ED with protection of personal freedom and civil liberty is one of the greatest challenges of civil commitment (Testa and West 2010). Although civil commitment may be lifesaving, a call has recently been made for legal regulations to minimize the harm associated with the psychological consequences of forced treatment (Tury et al. 2019).

Civil Commitment Around the World

Internationally, civil commitment laws range from strict legislation to none at all. Many Western countries use similar language in their civil commitment legislation, but specifics vary by region or state. The European Union legally permits compulsory admission of mentally ill persons only when a less restrictive environment might not be adequate or available. Compulsory admission is the intervention of last resort or applied only in an acute crisis or state of emergency. Criteria for civil commitment in the European Union are categorized into three groups. Serious threat of harm to self or others (dangerousness criterion) is an essential prerequisite for compulsory admission in Austria, Belgium, France, Germany, Luxembourg, and The Netherlands. Along with dangerousness, Italy, Spain, and Sweden use the need for psychiatric treatment as a crucial criterion for compulsory admission. Denmark, Finland, Greece, Ireland, Portugal, and the United Kingdom use a combination of serious mental disorder and dangerousness or serious mental disorder and need for treatment. The French do not stipulate a specific legal framework for civil commitment but have established two broad procedures: the first, known as *hospitalization d'office*, is executed by the police for persons with mental health problems who are considered a danger to public safety, and the second, *hospitalization à la demanded d'un tiers*, entitles family members or other close persons to apply to involuntarily place someone who may be unable to seek help him- or herself (Bowers 2014; de Stefano and Ducci 2008; Fennell and Goldstein 2006; Jacobsen 2012).

Germany, which has 16 federal states, independently organizes and regulates mental health care. Consequently, each federal state provides a separate legal framework for regulating involuntary placement or treatment of the mentally ill. Germany's basic philosophy emphasizes human rights as well as the self-determination of mentally ill patients and demands appropriate mental health care delivery in the least restrictive setting possible. This has generated a number of regulations or statutes across the federal states in an attempt to clarify or detail procedures for treating the mentally ill against their will. Nevertheless, despite the emphasis on need or right for treatment, the threat of harm to or by a mentally ill person is the crucial condition for civil commitment (Bowers 2014; de Stefano and Ducci 2008).

Countries that belong to the Commonwealth of Nations (a voluntary association of 53 sovereign states, nearly all of which were former British colonies or their dependencies) have very similar civil commitment legislation. Broadly, individuals may be admitted and detained as involuntary patients when they appear to be mentally ill. They must also need immediate treatment that they can only obtain by admission to and detention in an approved mental health service. Furthermore, due to mental illness, they are admitted and detained to protect their health or safety or that of the public. One may seek civil commitment of a person if that person, due to mental illness, refuses or is unable to consent to necessary treatment or could not receive adequate treatment in a less restrictive manner. In Australia, mental health law is constitutionally under state powers, with each state applying different laws. Consequently, some Australian states require that the person be a danger to society or self, whereas others only require that the person have a mental illness that needs treatment. Like Australia, New Zealand law requires that the person be a danger to self or others or be unable to care for him- or herself.

Every province and territory in Canada has legislation that permits individuals to be kept in a psychiatric hospital against their will. Two conditions must be satisfied: they must have a mental disorder or mental illness and must present a danger to themselves or others. If these two conditions are satisfied, the law authorizes a short period of assessment in a psychiatric facility. Generally, the assessment period is less than 72 hours, but patients may kept longer if two doctors indicate a need for continued assessment.

In the United Kingdom, legislation varies among different parts of the country, with England and Wales following one set of statues and Northern Ireland and Scotland providing their own laws. For England and Wales, all cases of civil commitment must be justified on the basis that the individual has a serious mental disorder and poses a risk of harm to self or others. Appropriate treatment must be available in the facility to which the person is being committed. In Scotland, patients with mental disorder (who are not capable of making decisions about their medical treatment) can be treated involuntarily. Under Northern Ireland law, the criteria for civil commitment require that the person have a mental disorder and that failure to detain would create a substantial likelihood of serious physical harm to the self or others (Bowers 2014; Fennell and Goldstein 2006).

Thus, civil commitment has similar or parallel definitions in the United States, the European Union, or former Commonwealth Nations. In most areas of the world, civil commitment laws focus on the concept of dangerousness to self or others. When a court upholds a finding of dangerousness, that person's right to refuse treatment ends. However, this broad understanding of civil commitment may be in trouble (Callaghan and Ryan 2014; Harpur 2012; U.N. General Assembly 2006). The U.N. Convention on the Rights of Persons with Disabilities (CRPD) directly contradicts civil commitment or involuntary treatment laws. The CRPD is an international treaty designed to protect the rights and dignity of all individuals with a disability, and mental illness is viewed as a disabling condition (U.N. General Assembly 2006). By October 2016, there were 160 signatories to this treaty from 167 states and the European Union. These nations affirmed that they will promote, protect, and ensure full enjoyment of human rights by persons with disabilities and acknowledge that all people with disabilities have full equality under the law as full and equal members of society (Callaghan and Ryan 2014; Harpur 2012; U.N. General Assembly 2006). The United States did not ratify this document and thus is not obligated to the CRPD (Callaghan and Ryan 2014; U.N. General Assembly 2006). This document states there is no place for involuntary treatment based on any disabling condition, including mental illness. Effectively, the United Nations has banned involuntary treatment (Callaghan and Ryan 2014; Harpur 2012; U.N. General Assembly 2006). By that reasoning, all states who signed the CRPD must revise their civil commitment laws; these new statutes would grant individuals with mental illness the same right to refuse treatment as those making decisions about medical care.

Civil Commitment in the United States

In the United States, all 50 states have statutes regarding civil commitment for psychiatric disorders. However, those statutes vary from state to state. In 8 states, the only ground for civil commitment is dangerousness, which means the person must demonstrate an immediate, physical danger to self or others before a court can intervene and order treatment. In the remaining 42 states, laws permit intervention based on an additional criterion that is broader than dangerousness to self or others, referred to as "grave disability" (Treatment Advocacy Center 2016). Although the exact wording varies, *grave disability* usually means a condition in which the individual, as a result of a mental disorder, is in danger of serious physical harm due to a failure to provide for his or her own essential human needs, such as food, clothing, or shelter. A person with a serious mental disorder who can voluntarily ask family, friends, or others to assist in meeting these needs does not fulfill this criterion. A third provision in which a court can intervene in a mental health crisis is called "need for treatment." Need-for-treatment standards (found in 26 states) include qualification for care based on at least one of the following conditions: 1) inability to obtain needed psychiatric care; 2) inability to make an informed medical decision; or 3) need for intervention to prevent further psychiatric or emotional deterioration (Treatment Advocacy Center 2016). While the extent of states' power to commit mentally ill persons on a "need for treatment" basis remains unclear, the U.S. Supreme Court allows the states considerable leeway in defining mental illness, danger to self or others, and gravely disabled (Treatment Advocacy Center 2016).

Evidentiary Standard for Civil Commitment in the United States

Although a civil process, involuntary treatment carries a heightened evidentiary standard of "clear and convincing evidence." This standard falls between the civil evidentiary standard of "preponderance of the evidence" and the criminal standard of "beyond a reasonable doubt." *Preponderance of the evidence* means "more likely than not" and applies to civil processes that do not traditionally involve fundamental civil liberties. *Beyond a reasonable doubt* is self-explanatory: each element of an alleged criminal offense must be proven beyond a reasonable doubt, given that the fundamental civil liberty of personal freedom is at issue.

Clear and convincing evidence is the civil standard first enunciated by the U.S. Supreme Court in the late 1970s in decisions involving persons with mental health disorders who were undergoing involuntary treatment (*Addington v. Texas* 1979). Clear and convincing evidence must be "free of substantial doubt." In a civil proceeding involving involuntary civil confinement for the treatment of mental health disorders, this means that the following must be proven by clear and convincing evidence: the patient with an ED has a mental health disorder, however that is defined in the state in which the action is brought, and as a result of having that mental health disorder, the patient is in need of involuntary treatment. This is usually couched in statutory language of whether the patient in question is dangerous to self or others and, in some jurisdictions, whether the patient is gravely disabled (unable to care for his or her essential needs).

Legal Definition of "Dangerousness"

The definition of what legally constitutes a patient with a mental health disorder being *dangerous* varies from state to state. Most states fall under the "umbrella" of one of three standards: the patient 1) has a "substantial probability" of becoming dangerous; 2) has a "substantial likelihood" of becoming dangerous; or 3) has a "substantial risk" of becoming dangerous. The first two standards are the most difficult to prove. The third legal standard of posing a "substantial risk" is the one most clearly aligned with the function of the mental health professional when evaluating someone with a mental health disorder. The mental health professional can perform a risk assessment of the patient in question and, in so doing, determine whether the he or she poses a "substantial risk" of engaging in dangerous behaviors, especially the longer that the patient is not engaged in treatment.

Grave Disability

Some states have a "gravely disabled" standard that allows people to be involuntarily hospitalized when they are unable to provide essential daily needs as a result of a mental health disorder. Both the mental health professional and the legal practitioner must understand not only the language of this particular definition but also the case law attendant to that standard.

Involuntary Use of Medications and Special Procedures

Authority to hospitalize a patient involuntarily does not necessarily equate with authority to administer medications or other treatments, such as nutrition for patients with EDs or electroconvulsive therapy for patients with severe depression (both of which are termed "special procedures"). Once the order for involuntary treatment is authorized, many states have a second "tier" to the process. Generally speaking, authority to involuntarily administer medications and nourishment must be granted either by a court that has jurisdiction, by state statutes, to hear evidence and decide whether involuntary treatment meets the state's standards or by an administrative panel empowered by statute with the same authority. The treatment standard varies from state to state, but it is generally couched as that the patient for whom involuntary treatment is sought be incapable of participating in or making informed decisions about the requested treatment due to the severity of his or her mental health disorder. Once that "hurdle" is cleared, standards generally require that the patient in question need the requested medication or special procedure to prevent harm befalling that patient or another person in the absence of the treatment being administered involuntarily. There may be yet an additional step of proving by clear and convincing evidence that the patient needs to have the treatment administered involuntarily to prevent long-term deterioration of his or her mental condition.

Most likely, clear and convincing evidence will also be needed that the benefits of administering the requested medication or special procedure clearly outweigh its potential risks and side effects. The fact finder, whether an administrative panel, court, or jury, will have to determine that no less drastic or invasive treatment alternatives are available to treat the severity of the person's mental health disorder. The fact finder will also have to engage in a balancing act of sorts to determine that all factors required by state statute or case law are proven by clear and convincing evidence.

Ethical Principles in the Civil Commitment of Individuals With Eating Disorders

Civil commitment as an approach to treatment for patients with EDs is not without its critics, controversies, or ethical concerns (Bowers 2018). Among the most debated ethical concerns are showing respect for patients' autonomy (allowing them to make their own decisions), nonmaleficence ("do no harm"), beneficence (providing care that benefits patients), and paternalism (interfering with patients' freedom for their own good). Each of these principles, as discussed in Chapter 2, adds a confounding dimension to the idea of involuntary treatment (Tansey 2011). An ethical dilemma arises between the autonomy of patients and beneficence. This is especially complicated when treating patients with EDs, which do not obviously or grossly impact their reality testing (Testa and West 2010). In this way, civil commitment involving a patient with AN differs from civil commitment of a patient with any other major psychiatric illness.

Gutheil and Bursztajn (1986) proposed several explanations for this. First, with AN, patients' lack of insight is confined to the narrow area of self-nutrition/body image rather than being pervasive and influencing multiple cognitive domains, as seen in those with schizophrenia or bipolar disorder who, by virtue of their severe psychotic or mood symptoms, are more obviously impaired. Second, the life-threatening nature of AN is often perceived not to be imminent. These patients usually present themselves well and are intelligent and articulate; they typically provide a rational explanation for their behavior and do not express an intent to die. Distinguishing an ED from culturally normative weight concerns can also be problematic, given media and social emphasis on thinness.

Despite these challenges in civilly committing patients with EDs, if their medical and psychiatric conditions meet the legal criteria for involuntary treatment, they should not be discounted from lifesaving treatment (Andersen 2007). Support of civil commitment indicates that the health care professional recognizes the severity of the ED, including its potential long-term impairment, and knows how hard it can be to alter the life-threatening course of illness. Civil commitment can be viewed as compassionate care. Short-term beneficence and paternalism trump autonomy in selected situations as long as autonomy is restored with treatment (Andersen 2007; Bowers 2014; Caplan 2006). The literature suggests that patients and their families experience relief (albeit temporarily) when accountability for care is transferred to the professional treatment team. This shift in responsibility from the family to the professional helps guide decision making about health that is distorted by the ED (Ramsay et al. 1999). In essence, it may be necessary to impose treatment (civil commitment) to save the life of the patient with a severe ED (Andersen 2007).

How Frequently Are Individuals With Eating Disorders Civilly Committed?

A relatively small proportion of the ED population is severely ill enough to be detained for treatment. Patients admitted involuntarily range from 1.5% to 11.6% in the United Kingdom (Elzakkers et al. 2014). Watson et al. (2000) indicated that 16.6% ($n=66$ of 397) of patients admitted to a hospital for specialized treatment warranted civil commitment. Data from other countries indicate a range from 8% (in Ireland) to 28% (in Australia). Specialized treatment programs civilly commit between 20% and 35% of their patients (Elzakkers et al. 2014).

Pros and Cons of Civil Commitment in Patients With Eating Disorders

Civil commitment is open to criticism because it strips people of their right to make autonomous decisions, even if the physician considers those decisions to be foolish. However, in hindsight, some patients have been thankful and seen their civil commitment as justified. This is especially true if the commitment was necessary to maintain the person's life and prevent serious medical problems and death (Guarda et al. 2007; Watson et al. 2000). Patients themselves have declared civil commitment as being important early in the course of treatment to prevent their disorder from becoming more chronic in nature (Guarda et al. 2007; Watson et al. 2000). However, patients treated involuntarily are often those who are more chronically ill and thus least likely to benefit from involuntary treatment. In a review of involuntary admission in patients with AN, Douzenis and Michopoulos (2015) noted involuntary treatment in these patients was most likely to be associated with three main indicators: the patient's past history (number of prior admissions), the complexity of the patient's condition (number of other psychiatric comorbidities), and the patient's current health risk (measured by BMI or risk of refeeding syndrome). Clausen et al. (2018) noted that the older the patient and the greater the number of comorbid psychiatric illnesses, the greater the likelihood of involuntary treatment.

The limited empirical data, though contradictory in nature, suggest involuntary treatment is beneficial at least in the short term (Andersen 2007). There is no difference in rate of weight restoration for involuntary versus voluntary patients (Brunner et al. 2005; Ramsay et al. 1999; Thiel and Paul 2007; Watson et al. 2000). However, in the long term, the outcome of patients treated on an involuntary basis may be worse than that of those treated voluntarily. This poor long-term outcome is not the result of civil commitment, per se, but rather because these patients have other validated poor prognostic factors (Ramsay et al. 1999). Involuntary tube feeding, although beneficial in the short term, may also confer a poor long-term prognosis (Elzakkers et al. 2014).

Patients' Perspective

A view from patients' perspective also suggests that the important aspect of civil commitment is not the involuntary treatment itself but how the person is treated during and after being civilly committed (Elzakkers et al. 2014; Tan et al. 2003). Any sense of coercion was related to the relationship between the patient and the mental health professional (Elzakkers et al. 2014; Tan et al. 2003). Although some patients saw civil commitment as a reason to continue engaging in treatment, others thought involuntary treatment should be reserved only for situations considered life threatening (Elzakkers et al. 2014; Tan et al. 2003). The timing of involuntary treatment is also imperative. Involuntary admission at a time when the patient is contemplating the need for change and recovery may, in fact, prove harmful for the patient's engagement in treatment (Douzenis and Michopoulos 2015). The context and relationships within which treatment decisions are made are critical to the patient's view of choice or compulsion for treatment. Freedom of choice is often less important than the relationships and attitudes of family members and health care workers. Some individuals see civil commitment as helpful and caring. Leverage or forced treatment can be deemed acceptable if the care provider and the patient have a shared and respected relationship (Tan and Richards 2015; Tan et al. 2003). The need for involuntary treatment is often perceived as coercive. However, this approach is validated by the serious nature of the ED. Paternalism or the perception of coercion need not endure long. Improvement in the patient's nutritional status can improve cognition and strengthen therapeutic alliance with the treatment team, leading to progress in treatment and a return of autonomy.

State Laws and Public Perception of Eating Disorders

Involuntary treatment of patients with EDs is still not a common occurrence in the United States. The public perception of a disorder such as AN in any given jurisdiction is most likely quite different from the reality. Most people are not aware of how deadly these disorders are or of the psychological consequences of malnutrition. Thus, it is highly likely that laws in many jurisdictions have "not caught up yet" to the realities of EDs. If the medical or legal professional is relatively new to this particular specialized area, it would serve him or her well to reach out to professionals in other jurisdictions who have experience presenting testimony in mental health proceedings in which the underlying diagnosis is an ED and involuntary treatment authority is requested. Colorado, Iowa, Maryland, and Minnesota are four jurisdictions where professionals have experience in dealing with ED cases requiring civil commitment.

Educating Attorneys and Fact Finders About the Severity of Eating Disorders

Legal professionals involved in these court commitment procedures must be aware that, although the patient with an ED may be highly functioning in many areas of life, the extreme dysfunction in this narrow spectrum can have catastrophic consequences when left untreated. The most direct way to educate the fact finder is to elicit testimony from the ED professional as to the significance of the severity of the patient's disorder. The fact finder will need to be educated in the following areas:

1. That the ED is a recognized mental health disorder in DSM-5 (American Psychiatric Association 2013);
2. That the ED has physical and mental manifestations in any individual;
3. That the human brain is an organ that needs proper nutrition, and that failure to provide nutrition will drastically negatively impact the brain's functioning;
4. That the best course of treatment is weight restoration, that the ability to provide nourishment involuntarily is critical for this particular patient to be weight restored, and that temporary weight restoration will not suffice; and
5. That the level of anxiety almost invariably rises with weight restoration.

The fact finder therefore must be shown that the best indicator of future behavior is past behavior. By the time a hearing occurs, the patient should have a well-documented history of treatment failure. It is critical to present as much detail as possible about past treatment episodes, including dates, lengths of stay, reasons for discharge, durations of time weight restoration was maintained, and repetitions of pattern on the patient's part.

Testimony of Family Members

Calling a patient's family members as witnesses in a hearing of this type can be a double-edged sword. Family members often have the best firsthand information about the patient's treatment history and attitude toward and cooperation with treatment and can provide the fact finder with specifics, such as how long the patient has been able to sustain weight gain before losing weight and falling back into the vicious grip of the ED. However, calling family members as witnesses has several potential pitfalls. The medical axiom of "first, do no harm" is a good starting point, ensuring that benefits of the family's testimony far outweigh any potential downsides. For example, if a family member's testimony revealed a power struggle between the person with ED and the family member testifying, such may diminish the severity of the ED in the fact finder's mind. The family's testimony must reflect genuine concern for the person with ED. If a dysfunctional dynamic comes out in the course of the testimony, such can lessen the impact of the family member's testimony.

Reviews and Appeals

A transcript will be the only record of the hearing regarding authorization for involuntary treatment. Given the confidential nature of mental health proceedings, video recording of the proceeding, wherein a reviewing body could see the physical condition of the patient for themselves, is highly unlikely. With this in mind, the legal professional must present evidence at each and every hearing as though that hearing will be appealed by the patient. The legal professional must fully understand that making a sound appellate record in an ED case is both different and likely more arduous than making a sound appellate record in a mental health hearing in which the underlying diagnosis is a psychotic disorder. Hearings regarding the involuntary treatment of a patient with an ED present a far more difficult puzzle for the legal professional to piece together for the administrative panel or judicial officer as well as the reviewing body or court. What may be apparent to the treatment professional and the legal professional will not necessarily be readily apparent to the reviewing court.

Case Law in the United States

As previously noted, each state has its own laws concerning civil commitment and the involuntary treatment of patients with psychiatric disorders. Courts in several states have applied these statutes with respect to the treatment of patients with EDs, and reviewing some of those decisions may be useful when considering involuntary treatment for a given patient. The courts have considered several important aspects about the treatment of patients with AN: the scope of the committing court in involving itself in treatment decisions (absent breach of standard of care), whether it is in the court's purview to agree that the patient is best served by receiving treatment in another state, that accurate criteria are used when presenting an argument for civil commitment, that the definition of grave disability does not necessitate the patient be close to death, and that medications may be warranted for treating patients with EDs. The cases discussed in the sections that follow were decided in the United States; cases regarding involuntary treatment versus futility can be found in Chapter 11.

In the Matter of Joanne Kolodrubetz

The first case calls into question the scope of a committing court in making treatment decisions. Ms. Kolodrubetz appealed a Minnesota District Court decision that denied her relief (*In the matter of Joanne Kolodrubetz* 1987). According to the Minnesota statute, the "committing court" only makes the initial legal determination as to whether a patient meets statutory criteria for commitment; once that determination has been made, the court will not review specific treatment modalities (with a few exceptions, such as electroconvulsive therapy). Patients who are challenging the specific form of treatment they are receiving must follow the Minnesota administrative review process.

Ms. Kolodrubetz presented to the Minnesota facility, where she was subsequently committed, with an extensive history of AN, to the degree that her life had been repeatedly endangered by her behaviors when she was not in treatment. She was civilly committed to the facility, but she did not agree with the treatment she received and pursued the administrative process. Unsatisfied by the findings and recommendations of that process, she then petitioned the court for relief. The appellate court determined that the Minnesota statutory process provided for involvement of the court only to the extent of making the initial determination of whether the patient met legal criteria for committal. Once the patient was committed, the facility's administrative process reviewed the efficacy of one treatment modality versus another. The court noted that it had "repeatedly stressed that the committing court may not involve themselves in treatment decisions" (*In the matter of Joanne Kolodrubetz* 1987) and that a patient who disagreed with the findings and recommendations of the administrative process should file a lawsuit seeking damages. The court also noted that the legal standard in such a lawsuit was "whether the treatment pursued by the facility was within accepted professional standards" (*In the Matter of Joanne Kolodrubetz* 1987).

In the Matter of Molly Kellor

Molly Kellor was initially committed to the University of Minnesota Hospital for a period of 6 months and subsequently committed for 12 months, with a plan to transfer her to a state psychiatric facility when she was medically stable. Ms. Kellor was transferred to the Willmar state facility, where she was partially weight-restored through tube feeding but gained little if any insight into her ED. She had a conflictual relationship with treatment staff at this facility, which was not a specialized ED treatment facility, and petitioned the court to transfer her to an out-of-state facility—Laureate, in Oklahoma—that specialized in ED treatment. The district court granted her request, finding that no in-state facilities in Minnesota offered ED-specific treatment and that, under Minnesota statute, Ms. Kellor was entitled to receive appropriate treatment in the least restrictive setting.

The People appealed this decision, basing their argument on the Minnesota statute, which, per *Kolodrubetz*, indicated the "committing court" only makes the initial legal determination as to whether the patient meets statutory criteria for commitment and does not review specific treatment modalities used at the facility. The appellate court held that the trial court (i.e., the committing court) has wide discretion in determining the least restrictive setting (*In the matter of Molly Kellor* 1994).

In re Judicial Commitment of W.R.

W.R., a 26-year-old female with AN, was admitted to a medical center in an emaciated state. She attempted to avoid caloric intake by discarding food, and she testified at her trial that she was eating too much and gaining weight too rapidly. The attending physician testified that W.R. had no insight into the severity of her mental condition, did not understand the need to take medication and undergo treatment, and could not provide for herself and would not survive if she were discharged. At trial, the responses given by W.R., who also had a psychotic illness, were described as "bizarre and not responsive to questions posed" (*In re Judicial Commitment of W.R.* 1994). In addition, although her parents provided testimony that reportedly reflected an awareness of their daughter's illness, they were noted as having failed to meet her needs in the past. W.R. appealed following a judgment that committed her for observation, care, and treatment of her mental illness. She argued that her commitment violated the due process clauses of the United States and Louisiana because, contrary to the trial judge's findings, she was not dangerous to herself or others and was capable of surviving safely in freedom with the help of willing family members. She also argued that the trial judge erred in finding that she was gravely disabled by clear and convincing evidence.

The higher court affirmed the trial court's decision, concluding that W.R.'s family had failed to meet her needs in the past and were unable to commit to providing her with the medical treatment she needed. The court also affirmed that "the evidence clearly and convincingly supports a finding that W.R. was gravely disabled as a result of her mental illness and is unable to survive safely in freedom" (*In re Judicial Commitment of W.R.* 1994).

In re S.A.M.

S.A.M. appealed an Iowa District Court decision determining that she met the definition of a person with a serious mental impairment and, as a result, was likely to inflict physical injury on herself or others if allowed to remain out of treatment. In filing the appeal, S.A.M. admitted that she had a mental illness, AN, and did not challenge the trial court's findings that she had serious mental impairment. However, S.A.M. challenged the trial court's finding of clear and convincing evidence that she was likely to inflict physical harm to herself if she were allowed to remain at liberty.

The reviewing court identified that the term "likely" in the statutory language was "construed to mean probable or reasonably to be expected." Given that S.A.M. had been able to maintain a stable body weight while in outpatient treatment just prior to being rehospitalized and had never had any metabolic abnormalities, even when at a lower body weight, the reviewing court determined that there was *not* clear and convincing evidence that it was "probable or reasonably expected" that she was likely to inflict physical injury upon herself if allowed to remain at liberty. Therefore, the trial court's ruling was reversed (*In re S.A.M.* 2005).

In re P.A.

P.A., who had a chronic and life-threatening ED, requested trials to the Denver Probate Court (*People of the State of Colorado in the interest of P.A.* 2012; *People of the State of Colorado in the interest of P.A.* 2013). In both cases, the court upheld the short-term certification for the statutory 3-month period, determining that P.A. was a danger to herself and gravely disabled. The probate court also granted the designated facility authority for both involuntary medication administration and involuntary feeding tube placement. P.A. appealed both decisions, alleging that because she had partially weight-restored in the facility (to which, on one of these occasions, she had weighed 43 lb at admittance), she was no longer gravely disabled or a danger to herself because she was no longer near death.

The appellate court found that "the definition of gravely disabled does not require that respondent be near death. Instead, it only requires that respondent be in danger of serious physical harm because of an inability or failure to provide one's self with the essential human needs of food and medical care" (*People of the State of Colorado in the interest of P.A.* 2012). The court specifically did not entertain whether P.A. was a danger to herself. P.A. also appealed the probate court order that granted involuntary administration of medications, asserting that the standard for involuntary medication set forth in *People v. Medina* (1985) had not been met by clear and convincing evidence. Involuntary administration of medication may be allowed if a physician or professional person shows by clear and convincing evidence that a patient is incompetent to effectively participate in treatment decisions; that treatment by medication is necessary to prevent significant and likely long-term deterioration in the patient's condition or the likelihood of the patient presenting serious harm to self or to others; that a less intrusive alternative is not available; and that the patient's need for treatment with the medication at issue is sufficiently compelling that it overrides her bona fide and legitimate concerns in refusing medication. Per the appellate court, P.A.'s mental illness had so impaired her judgment that she was incapable of participating in decisions affecting her health, and medication was needed to prevent the likelihood of her causing serious harm to herself, albeit indirectly. If she did not take medication, she would decompensate psychiatrically and (as a result) put herself in life-threatening danger by not taking in adequate nutrition. No less-viable alternatives were available to adequately treat her mental illness, because "anorexia nervosa is not conducive to non-medication therapies alone" (*People of the State of Colorado in the interest of P.A.* 2012) and (to that end), her psychiatrist testified that she would not be able to successfully treat P.A.'s AN without medication.

When P.A. appealed her certification again in 2013, it was her second appeal in a period of just over 1 year involving short-term commitment based on substantially similar circumstances. The court concluded that, based on these similar circumstances, the issues raised in the case were moot. Under the "mootness doctrine," an issue is moot when any judgment concerning it cannot have a practical effect on an existing controversy, and appellate courts will not render opinions on the merits of an appeal when the issues presented become moot because of subsequent events. According to the decision, "The fact the respondent is again before us under such similar circumstances supports our conclusion that the probate court's conclusion that she was gravely disabled at the time of the July 2013 is supported by sufficient evidence" (*People of the State of Colorado in the interest of P.A.* 2013).

In the interest of D.C.W.

On June 2, 2015, the Office of Mental Health and Intellectual Disabilities of Centre County, Pennsylvania, filed a petition to extend the involuntary treatment of the appellant, D.C.W., pursuant to section 7304 of the state's Mental Health Procedures Act. A mental health review officer conducted a hearing in which the treating psychiatrist testified that D.C.W. had AN, bingeing and purging type, that he had purged to the point of severe electrolyte abnormalities and dehydration and contraction alkalosis, and that his condition could lead to death, disability, or serious physical debilitation within 30 days. The appellant testified that he had been doing very well, was keeping his food down, and wanted to return home.

After the hearing, the mental health review officer granted the petition to extend the involuntary treatment for 90 days. D.C.W. then filed a petition for review of certification to the Centre County Court of Common Pleas. He argued that the state had failed to establish by clear and convincing evidence that he needed involuntary treatment when he was voluntarily working on techniques designed to abate his self-injurious behavior. The court disagreed, noting that for a person to be committed for an extended period of treatment it is not necessary to show that the patient committed an overt act within 30 days of the hearing, but it was necessary for the court to find that within the patient's most recent period of institutionalization that the patient's contact demonstrated a need for continuing involuntary treatment—that is, that his condition continued to show that he was a clear and present danger to himself or others. In considering the clear and convincing evidence standard, the court opined that the standards had been satisfied by the testimony of the staff psychiatrist and that "it was clear to this court that appellant was still in need of involuntary mental health treatment for his AN and without that treatment he had a reasonable probability of death, disability or serious debilitation within 30 days" (*In the interest of D.C.W.* 2016). The Superior Court thus affirmed that the trial court had properly certified the appellant's continued involuntary treatment based on the clear and present danger he presented to himself.

Conclusion

Civil commitment in ED treatment, although complicated in nature, is nonetheless worth considering for patients with severe and life-threatening EDs. There are pros and cons regarding the use of this form of involuntary treatment. Civil commitment may be damaging to the treatment relationship, and the patient may not view the treatment as necessary or lifesaving, even if that is the intent, although this is not always the case. Civil commitment laws vary around the world and from state to state, although in the United States the standard of proof can be no less than clear and convincing. Although further research into the use of civil commitment in these patients is needed, case law has informed our understanding of important legal questions and standards.

References

Addington v. Texas, 441 U.S. 418 (1979)

American Psychiatric Association: Treatment of Patients With Eating Disorders, 3rd Edition. Am J Psychiatry 163(7 suppl):4–54, 2006

American Psychiatric Association: Diagnostic and Statistical Manual of Mental Disorders, 5th Edition. Arlington, VA, American Psychiatric Association, 2013

Andersen A: Eating disorders and coercion. Am J Psychiatry 164:9–11, 2007

Anfang SA, Appelbaum PS: Civil commitment: the American experience. Isr J Psychiatry Relat Sci 43(3):209, 2006

Appelbaum PS: History of civil commitment and related reforms in the United States: lessons for today. Developments in Mental Health Law 25:13, 2006

Bloom JD: Thirty-five years of working with civil commitment statutes. J Am Acad Psychiatry Law 32(4):430–439, 2004

Bowers WA: Civil commitment in the treatment of eating disorders and substance abuse: empirical status and ethical considerations, in Eating Disorders, Addictions and Substance Use Disorders. Edited by Dennis AB. Berlin, Springer, 2014, pp 649–664

Bowers WA: Civil Commitment in the Treatment of Eating Disorders: Practical and Ethical Considerations. New York, Routledge, 2018

Brunner R, Parzar P, Resch F: Involuntary hospitalization of patients with anorexia nervosa: clinical issues and empirical findings. Fortschr Neurol Psychiatr 73:9–15, 2005

Callaghan SM, Ryan C: Is there a future for involuntary treatment in rights-based mental health law? Psychiatr Psychol Law 21(5):747–766, 2014

Caplan AL: Ethical issues surrounding forced, mandated or coerced treatment. J Subst Abuse Treat 31(2):117–120, 2006

Clausen L, Larsen JT, Bulik CM, Peterson L: A Danish based register study on involuntary treatment in anorexia nervosa. Int J Eat Disord 51:1213–1222, 2018

de Stefano A, Ducci G: Involuntary admission and compulsory treatment in Europe: an overview. Int J Ment Health 37(3):10–21, 2008

Douzenis A, Michopoulos I: Involuntary admission: the case of anorexia nervosa. Int J Law Psychiatry 39:31–35, 2015

Elzakkers IF, Danner UN, Hoek HW, et al: Compulsory treatment in anorexia nervosa: a review. Int J Eat Disord 47(8):845–852, 2014

Fennell P, Goldstein RL: The application of civil commitment law and practices to a case of delusional disorder: a cross-national comparison of legal approaches in the United States and the United Kingdom. Behav Sci Law 24(3):385–406, 2006

Guarda A, Pinto A, Coughlin J, et al: Perceived coercion and change in perceived need for admission in patients hospitalized for eating disorders. Am J Psychiatry 164:108–114, 2007

Gutheil TG, Bursztajn H: Clinicians' guidelines for assessing and presenting subtle forms of patient incompetence in legal settings. Am J Psychiatry 143:1020—1023, 1986

Harpur P: Embracing the new disability rights paradigm: the importance of the Convention on the Rights of Persons with Disabilities. Disabil Soc 27(1):1–14, 2012

In the interest of D.C.W., Sup. Court of Pennsylvania 2016 136.Ad 1027; 2016 WL 81798

In the matter of Joanne Kolodrubetz, 411 N.W. 2d 528 (Minn Ct. App. 1987)

In the matter of Molly Kellor, 520 N.W.2d 9 (Minn Ct. App. 1994)

In re Judicial Commitment of W.R., 649 So. 2d579 1994 LA App

In re S.A.M., 695 N. W. 2d 506 (Iowa App. 2005)

Jacobsen TB: Involuntary treatment in Europe: different countries, different practices. Curr Opin Psychiatry 25(4):307–310, 2012

People v. Medina, 705 P. 2d 961, 974 (Col 1985)

People of the State of Colorado in the interest of P.A., 12CA1024 (Col. App 2012)

People of the State of Colorado in the interest of P.A., 13CA1350 (Col. App 2013)

Ramsay R, Ward A, Treasure J, Russell GF: Compulsory treatment in anorexia nervosa: short-term benefits and long-term mortality. Br J Psychiatry 175(2):147–153, 1999

Tan J, Richards L: Legal and ethical issues in the treatment of really sick patients with anorexia nervosa, in Critical Care for Anorexia Nervosa: The MARSIPAN Guidelines in Practice. Edited by Robinson PH, Nicholls D. New York, Springer, 2015, pp 113–150

Tan JO, Hope T, Stewart A, Fitzpatrick R: Control and compulsory treatment in anorexia nervosa: the views of patients and parents. Int J Law Psychiatry 26(6):627–645, 2003

Tansey J: Ethical Analysis: Civil Commitment. Workshop presented at the 45th Association of Behavioral and Cognitive Therapy, Toronto, Canada, 2011

Testa M, West SG: Civil commitment in the United States. Psychiatry (Edgmont) 7:30–40, 2010

Thiel A, Paul T: Compulsory treatment in anorexia nervosa. Psychother Psychosom Med Psychol 57:128–135, 2007

Treatment Advocacy Center: State Standards for Assisted Treatment: Civil Commitment Criteria for Inpatient and Outpatient Psychiatric Treatment. Arlington, VA, Treatment Advocacy Center, 2016. Available at: https://www.treatmentadvocacycenter.org/browse-by-state. Accessed July 19, 2020.

Tury F, Szalai T, Szumska I: Compulsory treatment in eating disorders: control, provocation and the coercion paradox. J Clin Psychol 75(8):1444–1454, 2019

U.N. General Assembly: Convention on the Rights of Persons With Disabilities. 13 December 2006, A/RES/61/106, Annex 1

Watson TL, Bowers WA, Andersen AE: Involuntary treatment of eating disorders. Am J Psychiatry 157:1806–1810, 2000

Westmoreland P, Johnson C, Stafford M, et al: Involuntary treatment of patients with life-threatening anorexia nervosa. J Am Acad Psychiatry Law 45:419–425, 2017

7

Severe Eating Disorders in Children and Adolescents

How Are Childhood Eating Disorders Different?

Elizabeth Wassenaar, M.D.
Barbara Kessel, D.O.
Anne-Marie O'Melia, M.D.

Can We Diagnose Severe and Enduring Eating Disorders in Children and Adolescents?

Severe and enduring eating disorders (SEEDs) are defined as eating disorders (EDs) that last many years (3–10+) and are marked by severe medical and psychiatric pathology, significant use of resources, and poor outcomes (Hay and Touyz 2018; Robinson 2014). Problematic eating behaviors in early childhood often continue over time and can develop into full-fledged EDs (Marchi and Cohen 1990). As we recognize these disorders in younger and younger children, we are compelled to consider if we can or should apply the SEED criteria for patients who have an ED that is significant enough for long enough time to meet the criteria for a SEED to patients younger than 18. Currently, the topic of SEEDs in child and adolescent patients is a totally uncharted landscape with more questions than answers, including regarding its existence. Kaplan and Strober (2019) asked, "Is it possible to identify, soon after the illness begins, those who will maintain a severe, enduring illness course? Could early intervention prevent the development of severe and enduring illness? How young is too young for considering a palliative approach to treatment?" (p. 2).

Because we hypothesize that SEEDs in adult patients may be a unique entity, can we begin to identify children and adolescents who will develop a more severe form of the illness (Touyz and Hay 2015)? Data have shown that a shorter duration of illness is a promising sign for longer-term recovery (Franko et al. 2013). Would using the SEED paradigm in children and adolescents allow us to be more aggressive in implementing treatment interventions, and would identification of SEEDs in child or adolescent patients allow access to interventions that may change the course of their disorder? Is there benefit to using a chronic illness model to approach these patients—structuring long-term intervention and resources—or are we creating an exclusion criterion that makes it harder for them to receive care due to insurance limitations and resource constraints? How can we thoughtfully balance developmental concerns and tasks of childhood and adolescence with the treatment of SEEDs?

As we consider matters of involuntary treatment and palliative interventions for adults with SEEDs, adolescents with EDs begin to ask the same questions. But how young is too young for considering a palliative approach to treatment? In an article on euthanasia for anorexia nervosa (AN), "As Hard As It Gets: The Case of Anorexic E and the Right to Die," a young woman shared her story of making a request to die at age 18 after more than 5 years with severe AN: "A[t] the age of 18 I had a BMI of 10 kg/m² and was refusing all treatment, requesting I be allowed to die. At the time I truly felt that continuing was futile, I had spent years getting worse, not better" (Sokol 2012). Those of us who care for severely ill children and adolescents have surely heard a similar plea. Although mental illness does not qualify for physician-assisted death in the United States, nor is euthanasia available in this country, euthanasia is available for psychiatric illness and to minors in Belgium and The Netherlands. Children with chronic illness who are as young as 9 years have been allowed to end their lives in this manner (Deliens and van der Wal 2003; Samuel 2018; Securite de la Chaine Alimentaire et Environnement 2016).

In this chapter, we examine the current state of knowledge regarding the course of illness for children and adolescents with EDs and consider how these patients are compelled to receive treatment in cases when they may wish to refuse such care. In addition, we consider the special situation of transitional-age youths. Finally, we review the uncommon situation of factitious or imposed-factitious diagnoses of ED, including medical child abuse.

Course of Anorexia Nervosa in Children and Adolescents

AN has been clinically seen in patients from about age 7 onward. Although it presents similarly in children and adolescents compared with adults, some may have limited capacity for self-appraisal or reflection and may have difficulty putting their eating-disordered thoughts or feelings into words. For example, children may display similar eating-disordered behaviors but may not be able to voice their dissatisfaction with weight and shape (Nicholls and Bryant-Waugh 2009). Additionally, the physical impact on growth and developmental trajectories may be irreversible (Katzman 2005).

Data from a general practitioner register study reported an incidence of AN of 17.5 per 100,000 in 10- to 19-year-olds and 0.3 per 100,000 in 0- to 9-year-olds (Turnbull et al. 1996). Retrospective studies from the United States and Denmark have suggested that the illness affects a greater number of individuals (i.e., 9–27 per 100,000 for 10- to 14-year old girls and 3.7 per 100,000 for boys) (Joergensen 1992; Pfeiffer et al. 1986). The proportion of boys with childhood-onset AN is higher than in older adolescent samples, before the gender-specific effects of puberty have come into play.

Schoemaker (1997) noted the average time between onset of illness and admission to a treatment facility in six Western countries was 1.78 years for patients with AN. A study of 140 patients with AN ages 10–60 conducted in Germany by Neubauer et al. (2014) found a mean duration of untreated illness to be around 25.14 months. However, when broken down by age, there were significant differences in duration of illness prior to first treatment. A much longer duration of untreated illness, 38.35 months, was found in early onset AN (≤14 years of age) compared with 20.57 months in intermediate-onset AN (16–18 years) and 19.04 months in late-onset AN (≥19 years). In addition, that same study found that adolescents with EDs frequently presented with less desire for help and were 6.71 times more likely to be externally motivated for treatment than adults (Neubauer et al. 2014).

Binge Eating, Purging, and Bulimia Nervosa in Children and Adolescents

Although binge eating is reported as occurring in 6.2% of 6- to 13-year-olds, no reports have been made of bulimia nervosa (BN) in preadolescence. However, the literature does indicate that traits of childhood overeating are more common in women who later develop BN (Micali et al. 2007). Binge eating peaks in onset at 16–17 years, and the peak age at onset for purging is 17–18 years of age (Stice et al. 1998, 2009).

Utilizing data from the Western Australian Pregnancy Cohort (Raine) Study, which followed 2,868 children from pre-birth to 20 years old, Allen et al. (2013) assessed the course of early onset binge eating and purging disorders in a sample of 1,383 patients (49% of whom were male). Results of surveys from the participants at 14, 17, and 20 years of age indicated that 5.4% met full or partial criteria for binge eating disorder (BED), purging disorder, or BN at age 14, and a further 3.7% had subthreshold ED symptoms. The authors also noted that 19% of the 14-year-old subjects had experienced persistent BED, purging disorder, or BN until age 20; 44% achieved early remission (by age 17) without relapse; and a further 37% achieved later remission (by age 20). The likelihood of symptom remission in this cohort decreased over time. Although nearly half of the study subjects had achieved remission of their ED symptoms between 14 and 17 years of age, only one-third of the participants who met criteria for BED, purging disorder, or BN at 14 and 17 went into remission between the ages of 17 and 20. Participants with BED were more likely to have symptoms that persisted over a longer period of time and to transition to BN by age 17 (45%) (Allen et al. 2013).

Results of the Allen et al. (2013) study also indicated that participants who experienced persistent ED symptoms had higher degrees of externalizing behaviors, depressive symptoms, internalizing problems, and low self-esteem at age 17. Purging behaviors at age 17 and externalizing behaviors at age 14 were the strongest predictors of having a persistent ED at age 20. Furthermore, subjects with persistent ED pathology were less likely to finish high school and reported higher degrees of depression, anxiety, stress, and impairments in quality of life than those without. Finally, results of this study indicated that adolescents with a history of an ED continued to have greater-than-average subclinical ED symptoms and psychological distress compared with a control group. Early onset ED pathology can impact overall mental health and indicates risk for long-term impairments.

Treating Eating Disorders in Children and Adolescents

Recovery from AN in the short and long term cannot be achieved without interventions aimed at restoration of normal body weight (Stice et al. 2009; Steinhausen et al. 2009). The Maudsley Approach, also known as family-based treatment (FBT), has the most evidence to support its use in adolescents with EDs. Unlike more "traditional," individually based treatments, which tend to pathologize the family in the etiology of the ED, FBT considers parents a resource and essential to successful treatment for AN (Lock and Le Grange 2005). Manualized FBT takes place over the course of about 1 year, or 15–20 sessions that divide the treatment into three phases: phase I—weight restoration, phase II—returning control of eating back to the adolescent, and phase III—establishing a healthy adolescent identity (Lock 2001).

Studies of FBT have illustrated its efficacy. Approximately two-thirds of adolescent patients with AN are weight-recovered at the end of FBT, and 75%–90% are fully weight-recovered at 5-year follow-up (Eisler et al. 1997). Although little has been written regarding the best treatments for children and adolescents with BN, a recent randomized controlled trial conducted by Le Grange and his colleagues at the University of Chicago compared FBT with supportive psychotherapy and demonstrated that FBT may have promising results (Hail and Le Grange 2018).

Adolescent Rights and Ability to Refuse Care

The right of adolescents to seek or consent to mental health, substance abuse, or reproductive health care varies from state to state and internationally. In most of the United States, the age at which a minor becomes an adult, or age of majority, is 18 years. In other countries, the age of majority ranges from 14 to 21 years (Human Research Protection Office 2012; Kerwin et al. 2015). In many states, persons younger than 18 can consent to receive treatment as mature minors without parental involvement; however, parents may still compel their minor child into involuntary care. However, some states, statutes require that minors consent to receive treatment (Kerwin et al. 2015). In select cases, the courts have upheld the rights of minors to refuse lifesaving interventions. However, in these cases, mental illness was not a consideration (Craig 2015; Skeels 2016; WCVB Boston 2012). Families facing these issues must become familiar with the laws in their state and the resources available in the event that their minor child refuses lifesaving interventions and they need to pursue legal determination of incompetency to make these sorts of medical decisions (Fortunati et al. 2006; National Conference of State Legislatures 2019).

The right to consent to or refuse treatment is a separate concern from the right for confidentiality in treatment. The type of information and the age at which a minor may direct confidentiality also varies among states (Morreale et al. 2005). This can be concerning to parents whose children wish to withhold important information about their treatment, including their health status and interventions. Physicians often discuss the limits of confidentiality with their minor patients, including risk to self or others, in cases of abuse, neglect, or sexual activity involving minors younger than the age of consent (U.S. Department of Health and Human Services 2015). Establishing and maintaining relationships with physicians and specialists in treating EDs can assist families strategize how best to work with the information they do have to support their child.

Treating Transitional-Age Youth With Eating Disorders

Transitional-age youth, or emerging adult-age patients, are increasingly being carved out from adolescent and adult patient populations because of the specific challenges and needs of this particular population. Transitional-age youth are people between the ages of 16 and 25 years who are in a stage of immense change, with significant life transitions and developmental tasks (Munsey 2006). In this time, young people typically move from their primary families into the larger world of postsecondary education, work, and starting families of their own; they are considered adults in the eyes of the law, can legally purchase addictive substances, and begin to age out of the pediatric health care system. Parenting a young adult is its own developmental phase, with renegotiation of the parent–child relationship and increased autonomy for parents. Parenting a young adult with a serious medical or psychiatric condition introduces unique challenges. Developmental tasks of young adulthood are often put on hold and can remain in moratorium for years, especially in the cases of uncertain disease course and possibility of recovery (Rolland 1987).

FBT is generally viewed as the treatment of choice for children and adolescents with EDs, in combination with medical stabilization and nutritional rehabilitation (Fisher et al. 2018). FBT for transitional-age youth has been introduced as a hybrid approach for young adults with EDs and emphasizes collaboration and age-appropriate autonomy. Family therapy has limited data in more severe cases but has shown promise in severely ill adolescents with AN (Fink et al. 2017). In adults with SEED-AN, cognitive-behavioral therapy and specialist-supportive clinical management show modest improvements in BMI and quality of life (Robinson 2014).

Medical Child Abuse

Factitious disorder is a psychiatric diagnosis in which patients impose symptoms or misrepresent illness or injury for various reasons, including maintaining relationships with treatment providers. When evaluating SEEDs in children, especially patients with confounding symptoms, be sure to consider factitious disorder imposed on another. Caregiver-fabricated illness is relatively rare but can present in patients with gastrointestinal symptoms, including malnutrition, food allergies and reactions, and gastrointestinal surgeries. Although in many of these cases the child is very young, at least 25% of cases reported have been investigated in children older than 6 years of age, and notable cases in older children and adolescents have been reported (Ali-Panzarella et al. 2017; Faedda et al. 2018; Rabago et al. 2015).

In situations in which suspicion arises for factitious presentation, coordinate with other providers to collect inconsistencies. Sometimes, covert surveillance can be used while the child is hospitalized. Factitious disorder imposed on another is a form of abuse, and child protective services should become involved when sufficient data support this diagnosis (Flaherty et al. 2013).

Conclusion

The concept of SEEDs in a young patient population raises difficult and important theoretical and ethical discussions. As we learn more about the disease process and diagnostic understanding of EDs, we will enhance our ability to understand why some disorders become SEEDs and to tailor interventions that can prevent long-term morbidity and mortality.

References

Ali-Panzarella AZ, Bryant TJ, Marcovitch H, Lewis JD: Medical child abuse (Munchausen syndrome by proxy): multidisciplinary approach from a pediatric gastroenterology perspective. Curr Gastroenterol Rep 19(4):14, 2017

Allen KL, Byrne SM, Oddy WH, Crosby RD: Early onset binge eating and purging eating disorders: course and outcome in a population-based study of adolescents. J Abnorm Child Psychol 41(7):1083–1096, 2013

Craig AE: Diazepam discord: a competent minor's constitutional right to seek and refuse psychotropic medication. Journal of Legislation 41(1):103–125, 2015

Deliens L, van der Wal G: The euthanasia law in Belgium and The Netherlands. Lancet 362(9391):1239–1240, 2003

Eisler I, Dare C, Russell GF, et al: Family and individual therapy in anorexia nervosa: a 5-year follow-up. Arch Gen Psychiatry 54(11):1025–1030, 1997

Faedda N, Baglioni V, Natalucci G, et al: Don't judge a book by its cover: factitious disorder imposed on children. Report on 2 cases. Front Pediatr 6:110, 2018

Fink K, Rhodes P, Miskovic-Wheatley J, et al: Exploring the effects of a family admissions program for adolescents with anorexia nervosa. J Eat Disord 3(suppl 1):O48, 2017

Fisher CA, Skocic S, Rutherford KA, Hetrick SE: Family therapy approaches for anorexia nervosa. Cochrane Database Syst Rev 10:CD004780, 2018

Flaherty EG, MacMillan HL, Committee on Child Abuse and Neglect: caregiver-fabricated illness in a child: a manifestation of child maltreatment. Pediatrics 132(3):590–597, 2013

Fortunati F, Morgan CA, Temporini H, et al: Juveniles and competency to stand trial. Psychiatry (Edgmont) 3(3):35–38, 2006

Franko DL, Keshaviah A, Eddy KT, et al: Do mortality rates in eating disorders change over time? A longitudinal look at anorexia nervosa and bulimia nervosa. Am J Psychiatry 170(8):917–925, 2013

Hail L, Le Grange D: Bulimia nervosa in adolescents: prevalence and treatment challenges. Adolesc Health Med Ther 9:11–16, 2018

Hay P, Touyz S: Classification challenges in the field of eating disorders: can severe and enduring anorexia nervosa be better defined? J Eat Disord 6:41, 2018

Human Research Protection Office: Determining the Legal Age to Consent to Research. St. Louis, MO, Washington University, 2012. Available at: https://hrpo.wustl.edu/wp-content/uploads/2015/01/5-Determining-Legal-Age-to-Consent.pdf. Accessed April 4, 2019.

Joergensen J: The epidemiology of eating disorders in Fyn County, Denmark, 1977–1986. Acta Psychiatr Scand 85(1):30–34, 1992

Kaplan AS, Strober M: Severe and enduring anorexia nervosa: can risk of persisting illness be identified, and prevented, in young patients? Int J Eat Disord 52(4):478–480, 2019

Katzman DK: Medical complications in adolescents with anorexia nervosa: a review of the literature. Int J Eat Disord 37(suppl):S52–S59, discussion S87–S89, 2005

Kerwin ME, Kirby KC, Speziali D, et al: What can parents do? A review of state laws regarding decision making for adolescent drug abuse and mental health treatment. J Child Adolesc Subst Abuse 24(3):166–176, 2015

Lock J: Treatment Manual for Anorexia Nervosa: A Family Based Approach. New York, Guilford, 2001

Lock J, Le Grange D: Help Your Teenager Beat an Eating Disorder. New York, Guilford, 2005

Marchi M, Cohen P: Early childhood eating behaviors and adolescent eating disorders. J Am Acad Child Adolesc Psychiatry 29(1):112–117, 1990

Micali N, Holliday J, Karwautz A, et al: Childhood eating and weight in eating disorders: a multi-centre European study of affected women and their unaffected sisters. Psychother Psychosom 76(4):234–241, 2007

Morreale MC, Stinnett AJ, Dowling EC (eds): Policy Compendium on Confidential Health Services for Adolescents, 2nd Edition. Chapel Hill, NC, Center for Adolescent Health and the Law, 2005. Available at: http://www.cahl.org/PDFs/PolicyCompendium/PolicyCompendium.pdf. Accessed April 4, 2019.

Munsey C: Emerging adults: the in-between age. Monitor on Psychology 37(7):68, 2006

National Conference of State Legislatures: Juvenile Justice: States With Juvenile Competency Laws. Washington, DC, National Conference of State Legislatures, 2019. Available at: http://www.ncsl.org/research/civil-and-criminal-justice/states-with-juvenile-competency-laws.aspx. Accessed April 4, 2019.

Neubauer K, Weigel A, Daubmann A, et al: Paths to first treatment and duration of untreated illness in anorexia nervosa: are there differences according to age of onset? Eur Eat Disord Rev 22(4):292–298, 2014

Nicholls D, Bryant-Waugh R: Eating disorders of infancy and childhood: definition, symptomatology, epidemiology, and comorbidity. Child Adoles Psychiatr Clin North Am 18(1):17–30, 2009

Pfeiffer RJ, Lucas AR, Ilstrup DM: Effect of anorexia nervosa on linear growth. Clin Pediatr 25(1):7–12, 1986

Rabago J, Marra K, Allmendinger N, Shur N: The clinical geneticist and the evaluation of failure to thrive versus failure to feed. Am J Med Genet 169(4):337–348, 2015

Robinson P: Severe and enduring eating disorders: recognition and management. Adv Psychiatr Treat 20(6):392–401, 2014

Rolland JS: Chronic illness and the life cycle: a conceptual framework. Family Process 26(2):203–221, 1987

Samuel H: Belgium authorised euthanasia of a terminally ill nine and 11-year-old in youngest cases worldwide. The Telegraph, August 7, 2018. Available at: https://www.telegraph.co.uk/news/2018/08/07/belgium-authorised-euthanasia-terminally-nine-11-year-old-youngest. Accessed January 11, 2019.

Schoemaker C: Does early intervention improve the prognosis in anorexia nervosa? A systematic review of the treatment-outcome literature. Int J Eat Disord 21(1):1–15, 1997

Securite de la Chaine Alimentaire et Environnement: Euthanasie: Médecins. SPF Brussels, Belgium, Santé Publique, 2016. Available at: https://www.health.belgium.be/fr/sante/prenez-soin-de-vous/debut-et-fin-de-vie/euthanasie/euthanasie-medecins. Accessed April 4, 2019.

Skeels JF: In re E.G.: the right of mature minors in Illinois to refuse lifesaving medical treatment. Summer 1990 Health Law Symposium 21(4):1199–1230, 2016

Sokol D: 'As hard as it gets': the case of anorexic E and the right to die. The Guardian, June 19, 2012

Steinhausen H-C, Grigoroiu-Serbanescu M, Boyadjieva S, et al: The relevance of body weight in the medium-term to long-term course of adolescent anorexia nervosa: findings from a multisite study. Int J Eat Disord 42(1):19–25, 2009

Stice E, Killen JD, Hayward C, Taylor CB: Age of onset for binge eating and purging during late adolescence: a 4-year survival analysis. J Abnorm Psychol 107(4):671–675, 1998

Stice E, Marti CN, Shaw H, Jaconis M: An 8-year longitudinal study of the natural history of threshold, subthreshold, and partial eating disorders from a community sample of adolescents. J Abnorm Psychol 118(3):587–597, 2009

Touyz S, Hay P: Severe and enduring anorexia nervosa (SE-AN): in search of a new paradigm. J Eat Disord 3(1):26, 2015

Turnbull S, Ward A, Treasure J, et al: The demand for eating disorder care: an epidemiological study using the general practice research database. Br J Psychiatry 169(6):705–712, 1996

U.S. Department of Health and Human Services: Statutory Rape: A Guide to State Laws and Reporting Requirements. Washington, DC, U.S. Department of Health and Human Services, 2015. Available at: https://aspe.hhs.gov/report/statutory-rape-guide-state-laws-and-reporting-requirements. Accessed April 4, 2019.

WCVB Boston: Teen who ran from chemo 18 years ago now cancer-free. WCVB Boston, April 3, 2012. Available at: https://www.wcvb.com/article/teen-who-ran-from-chemo-18-years-ago-now-cancer-free/8169155. Accessed April 4, 2019.

8

Novel Treatments for Patients With Severe and Enduring Eating Disorders

Leah Brar, M.D.
Elizabeth Wassenaar, M.D.
Anne-Marie O'Melia, M.D.

TREATING individuals with eating disorders (EDs) is a complex endeavor. Nutrition is the mainstay of treatment but is seldom sufficient by itself. Once a person has begun the weight restoration process, psychotherapy is imperative, although cognitive-behavioral therapy and family therapy have been found to be most effective in people who are weight-restored (Yager et al. 2010). Individuals who are younger, have a shorter duration of illness, and achieve full weight restoration typically have the most favorable prognosis (Accurso et al. 2014; Hetman et al. 2017). However, little consensus has been found as to what types of treatment might be successful in patients with severe unremitting EDs (Touyz et al. 2013). Such patients, regarded as having severe and enduring eating disorders (SEEDs), have failed to respond to treatment with full weight restoration, are typically ill for a decade or longer, and are often as debilitated as patients diagnosed with severe mental illnesses such as bipolar disorder or schizophrenia. Although patients with SEEDs are often prescribed medications and undertake psychotherapy for comorbid depression, anxiety, and PTSD, little assuages the symptoms of the ED itself. Touyz and Hay (2015) noted that patients with SEEDs "have suffered far too long, having to contend with an abysmal quality of life, devoid of any hope of an effective treatment on the horizon" (Touyz and Hay 2015). ED treatment professionals and researchers alike have therefore investigated the use of novel, off-label treatments. In this chapter, we review novel pharmacological interventions, neuromodulatory treatments, surgical options, and complementary and alternative medicine interventions for these patients.

Pharmacological Interventions

Anorexia Nervosa, Restricting Type

Currently, no medications are FDA approved for the treatment of anorexia nervosa (AN). Evidence supporting the efficacy of pharmacotherapy has been limited thus far. Antidepressants have not been demonstrated to be effective in treating the primary symptoms of AN (Aigner et al. 2011). The role of second-generation antipsychotics has been explored with mixed results (McElroy et al. 2015b). One review of randomized placebo-controlled trials indicated olanzapine may have the best evidence overall but noted limitations related to small sample size in the included studies. The authors theorized that certain AN subpopulations might be more responsive to second-generation antidepressants, such as patients with prominent anxiety and obsessive-compulsive symptoms.

The results of a chart review of nine patients with severe, treatment-resistant AN whose body image distortion reached delusional proportions indicated that low doses of haloperidol reduced body image disturbance and drive for thinness (Mauri et al. 2013). The patients in this review all had BMIs <13 kg/m^2 and were treated in an inpatient setting. Although antipsychotic medications may indeed reduce the anxiety related to body image distortion, it is nonetheless important to recognize that they may have untoward side effects. Their QTc-prolonging effect should not be underestimated in patients with low BMI, especially those with the purging form of AN and its resulting electrolyte-imbalance QTc-prolonging actions (Westmoreland et al. 2016). The long-term side effects of antipsychotics, such as tardive dyskinesia, to which women are especially prone, should also be considered. A randomized, double-blind, placebo-controlled crossover study on the effects of alprazolam in a laboratory test meal revealed no significant increases in caloric intake or anxiety, indicating a limited role for the medication in AN (Steinglass et al. 2014).

Several studies have examined the potential role of hormones in the treatment of AN. Ghrelin (a hormone produced and released mainly by the stomach) has been termed the "hunger hormone" because it stimulates appetite, increases food intake, and promotes fat storage. A small randomized, double-blind, placebo-controlled clinical trial of relamorelin (an agonist of ghrelin) in the outpatient setting demonstrated decreases in gastric emptying time and weight gain after only 4 weeks (Fazeli et al. 2018).

Another study indicated that administration of dehydroepiandrosterone, an endogenous steroid produced in the adrenal glands that functions as a precursor to sex hormone production, resulted in an increase in BMI without an increase in bone mineral density (Bloch et al. 2012). Transdermal estradiol decreased trait anxiety but had no effects on eating or body image compared with placebo in a study of adolescent girls with AN (Misra et al. 2013). Oxytocin, a peptide hormone released by the posterior pituitary with roles in sexual reproduction and bonding, has also been studied; one study showed reductions in attentional biases toward eating-related stimuli and negative shape stimuli following a single dose of intranasal oxytocin in a laboratory setting, an effect that correlated with autistic spectrum traits. However, it had no effect on caloric intake (Kim et al. 2014). Another placebo-controlled trial of daily oxytocin for 4–6 weeks in the inpatient setting also demonstrated no changes in weight but reduced eating concern and cognitive rigidity when compared with placebo (Russell et al. 2018).

Tyrosine, an essential amino acid and precursor to catecholamines that may affect cognitive functioning, has been studied. A double-blind, randomized crossover trial of tyrosine supplementation for 3 weeks in 19 hospitalized females with AN indicated shortened reaction times in tests of memory and improvements in depressed mood, suggesting a potential role for the amino acid in improving cognitive functioning in AN (Israely et al. 2017).

The use of cannabis as a panacea for symptoms of mental illness is highly controversial. Although medical and recreational use of cannabis is legal in many states, this has not translated into treatment for psychiatric symptoms that is free from side effects, and few randomized controlled trials to this effect are available. One study using dronabinol revealed a small but significant improvement in weight gain when compared with placebo (Andries et al. 2014). In contrast, low doses of Δ^9-tetrahydrocannabinol over 1 month revealed significant improvements in psychological symptoms, such as depression and ascetism, without significant changes in BMI (Avraham et al. 2017). Significant side effects must be considered when evaluating the usefulness of cannabis in patients with SEEDs. Considerable evidence shows that cannabis impacts the risk of psychosis, especially when used during adolescence (Mustonen et al. 2018; Volkow et al. 2016). Cannabis use has also been associated with cyclic vomiting syndrome, which is a syndrome of recurrent incapacitating nausea and vomiting, and with cannabis hyperemesis syndrome, which is associated with cessation of cannabis use, recurrent nausea and vomiting, and abdominal pain. Vomiting syndromes could both precipitate eating-disordered behaviors and compromise health, making these two entities especially dangerous to patients with SEEDs (Bajgoric et al. 2015; Pattathan et al. 2012).

Ketamine, an anesthetic agent, has demonstrated efficacy as a rapidly acting antidepressant agent in patients whose illness had not responded to other treatment trials (Rotroff et al. 2016). A study of female mice administered a single injection of ketamine in midadolescence found that subjects experienced increased food intake and weight gain during recovery when subsequently exposed to activity-based AN. Furthermore, a small cohort of patients with refractory EDs showed reductions in compulsivity and normalization of weight (Mills et al. 1998).

Bulimia Nervosa

Fluoxetine is the only medication approved by the FDA for the treatment of bulimia nervosa (BN). Studies involving potential novel treatments are rare. Erythromycin, chosen for study due to its prokinetic effects on gastric emptying, demonstrated no significant clinical benefits after 6 weeks when compared with placebo (Devlin et al. 2012). An internet survey of patients with BN or binge eating disorder (BED) regarding the efficacy of baclofen (a GABA$_B$ agonist with anecdotal evidence for reducing ED behaviors) indicated potential positive effects, although the authors acknowledged a potential selection bias because the patients who experienced improvements might have been more likely to respond to the survey (Imbert et al. 2017). In addition, acute psychosis was described in one patient treated for BED, affirming the need for controlled evaluation of this medication (Ricoux et al. 2019).

Ayahuasca is a psychoactive plant-based tea used for medical and spiritual reasons by indigenous groups in the Amazon. Its use in the treatment of symptoms related to trauma and substance addiction is being investigated. The hallucinogenic effect of this psychoactive substance results from N,N-dimethyltryptamine, which is currently a Schedule I controlled substance in the United States (meaning it is classified as having no medical use and a high potential for abuse; U.S. Drug Enforcement Administration 2019). However, the effects of ayahuasca on addiction are being studied in other countries (Ricoux et al. 2019; Thomas et al. 2013). Interviews with people previously diagnosed with EDs who independently participated in ceremonial ayahuasca revealed themes of reduced ED symptoms and body concerns as well as improved ability to process painful emotional content.

Part of the ceremonial use of ayahuasca involves a "purge," and participants reported that this component was not triggering to their ED. To date, only patients with a history of AN or BN have been interviewed (Lafrance et al. 2017; Ricoux et al. 2019).

Binge Eating Disorder

Lisdexamfetamine is currently the only agent approved by the FDA for the treatment of BED. However, several medications have been examined as potential off-label alternatives. According to a case report, naltrexone monotherapy dosed at 100 mg/day led to a reduction in binge-eating episodes and a 3-kg weight loss in a male patient with comorbid BED and alcohol use disorder (Leroy et al. 2017). Combination naltrexone extended-release and bupropion extended-release therapy resulted in increased control of eating, reduced weight, and ameliorated depressive symptoms in 25 women with both BED and major depressive disorder (Guerdjikova et al. 2017). Nalmefene, an opioid receptor modulator used in Europe for reducing problematic alcohol use, resulted in elimination of binge eating in a case report (Marazziti et al. 2016).

An open-label, prospective study of combined phentermine and topiramate therapy produced associations with reduced binge-eating frequency and weight (Guerdjikova et al. 2018). Patients given chromium (an essential mineral that directly enhances insulin) in varying doses over 6 months experienced dose-dependent reductions in fasting glucose but no statistically significant differences in binge frequency or body weight (Brownley et al. 2013). A double-blind trial of oxytocin demonstrated no statistically significant reductions in binge-eating episodes compared with placebo (Agabio et al. 2016).

A case report of an adolescent male with autism, comorbid food cravings, and weight gain indicated that 36 weeks of treatment with liraglutide, a glucagon-like peptide-1 analogue, was well tolerated and resulted in decreased cravings and compulsive eating, with a 12% reduction in weight (Järvinen et al. 2019). In a rat model in which non-food-deprived rats were offered limited access to optional dietary fat (lard) in additional to normal chow to mimic binge eating, researchers found a potential role for glutamatergic neurotransmission in obesity and disordered eating (Popik et al. 2011). The researchers demonstrated that sibutramine decreased lard consumption and increased chow consumption, but these effects disappeared after treatment. Memantine (an NMDA antagonist that inhibits excessive glutamate release) and an mGluR5 antagonist both caused similar effects that persisted after treatment, but only memantine produced statistically significant intake differences (Johnson and Kotermanski 2006).

An open-label, prospective, flexible-dose study of sodium oxybate, which is an analogue for GABA, an inhibitory neurotransmitter, in BED reported that 9 of 12 participants had remission of binge eating over 16 weeks and that 5 participants lost more than 5% of their baseline weight (McElroy et al. 2011). A randomized, placebo-controlled trial of armodafinil, which works in the dopaminergic system, resulted in a statistically higher rate of decreased binge frequency over 10 weeks (McElroy et al. 2015a).

Neurostimulation

Neurostimulation has been defined as any intervention intended to alter nervous system function using energy fields such as electricity, magnetism, or both (Dalton et al. 2018a). Such interventions include transcranial magnetic stimulation (TMS), electroconvulsive therapy (ECT), and deep brain stimulation (DBS). These interventions vary in their invasiveness and propensity for side effects. Given that individuals with SEED are often physically frail, the physical condition of the patient for whom the therapy is being considered must be carefully evaluated. Examples include cardiac status in preparation for general anesthetic for ECT, risk of infection or stroke with implantation of DBS simulator, and propensity to develop delirium as a result of all three therapies. Ethical and legal concerns might also arise with regard to whether a person with a severe ED has the ability to consent to such treatment, especially when the treatment in question is relatively untested in these disorders and is invasive or confers a high likelihood of side effects.

Transcranial Magnetic Stimulation

TMS is a noninvasive neuromodulatory treatment for severe mental illness. Initially approved for treatment-resistant depression, it is now being evaluated for efficacy in other mental illnesses, including OCD and autism spectrum disorder. Repetitive TMS (rTMS) delivers magnetic pulses to specific areas of the brain and has been shown to potentially change cortical activity and increase neuroplasticity. Low frequencies inhibit the areas being targeted, whereas higher frequencies (>5 Hz) activate targeted regions (Dalton et al. 2017). In EDs, because effective treatment interventions have been limited, rTMS is being evaluated as a viable option for the most severely ill patients. It is promising because it does not require compliance with daily medication, is a time-limited intervention, and is not contingent on weight restoration for efficacy. Initial evidence for the treatment of AN with TMS has been encouraging. The Transcranial Magnetic Stimulation and Neuroimaging in Anorexia Nervosa study found positive changes in mood, obsessive-compulsive symptoms, and quality-of-life scores in individuals with severe and enduring AN (Dalton et al. 2018b). Although only small changes in ED symptoms or BMI were found in the 4-month study time frame, both measures also favored rTMS intervention. Other studies have found decreases in anxiety, feeling of being fat, or overfullness (Van den Eynde et al. 2013).

Deep TMS targets the insula as a novel target based on observations that insular dysfunction may be a key component of AN. The insula combines visual and bodily perceptions, regulates awareness of positive and negative feelings, and inhibits higher-order cognitive functions. Using a Hased coil, daily treatments on a small group of underweight (mean BMI 16.6) women with SEEDs for up to 6 weeks demonstrated changes in ED-related obsessions and compulsions. Persistent results were observed up to 6 months posttreatment (Knyahnytska et al. 2019). In addition, patients with nonspecific diagnoses of an ED (AN, BN, ED not otherwise specified) and PTSD showed improvements in emotional regulation following TMS treatment targeting the dorsomedial prefrontal cortex, a novel target associated with self-control that shows more abnormalities on PTSD neuroimaging studies (Woodside et al. 2017). Case reports of rTMS targeting the dorsomedial prefrontal cortex in patients with BN demonstrated remission in all ED symptoms, and larger studies showed a decrease in bingeing behaviors but not consistently in purging behaviors (Downar et al. 2012; Walpoth et al. 2008). In obese patients without identified BED, rTMS decreased calorie intake and impacted weight loss in just four sessions over 2 weeks (Kim et al. 2018). Trials of the efficacy of TMS in patients with BED are ongoing (Maranhão et al. 2015).

Transcranial direct current stimulation (tDCS) delivers weak electrical current to brain regions through electrodes placed on the scalp in order to either depolarize (anodal tDCS) or hyperpolarize (cathodal tDCS) target regions (Thair et al. 2017) Typically, the dorsolateral prefrontal cortex on the right or left is targeted (Forcano et al. 2018). Evidence for use of tDCS in EDs is limited; to date, studies have looked at tDCS for binge eating and bulimia, and promising results have been found in OCD (Brunelin et al. 2018; Forcano et al. 2018; Kekic et al. 2017). Cranial electrotherapy stimulation, including "alpha-stim" devices or Fisher Wallace stimulators, delivers weak, alternating pulsed electrical current through battery-powered sponge electrodes. It was developed for insomnia, with some applications in depression, anxiety, and pain management; to date, no data are available regarding its use in EDs and little information is available on the potential side effects it may have on patients with medical complications related to severe EDs (Horowitz 2013).

Deep Brain Stimulation

DBS involves a neurosurgical procedure in which electrodes are implanted in an individual's brain. Once the electrodes are activated, electrical pulses are delivered to targeted brain structures in the limbic system and limbic pathway, such as the cingulate cortex and the nucleus accumbens (which targets areas of suspected dysfunction related to reward and mood), given evidence for the involvement of these brain structures in refractory movement disorders and OCD (Lozano et al. 2019). The electrodes can be activated as soon as surgery is completed but often require months to optimize the effect. In EDs, DBS has been investigated in severe and enduring AN. DBS was first recorded as an intervention for severe refractory AN in 2011 (Lipsman et al. 2013). More recently, 16 patients with refractory AN underwent DBS and reported improvements in weight, mood, and anxiety and changes in cerebral glucose metabolism in regions of the brain associated with disease, including the insular area involved in interoception, the parietal regions involved in body perception, the anterior cingulate gyrus involved in affect regulation, and temporal regions involved in social cognitive behavior (Lipsman et al. 2017). Furthermore, targeting the nucleus accumbens, which is involved in the regulation of food intake, has been demonstrated to impact appetite signaling in both hypo- and hyperphagia, which may have implications in the treatment of severe and enduring AN (Park et al. 2018; Prinz and Stengel 2018; Whiting et al. 2013).

Electroconvulsive Therapy

ECT involves inducing a cerebral seizure in an anesthetized patient. A valuable treatment intervention for severe depression, bipolar disorder, psychosis, and catatonia (Salik and Marwaha 2019), ECT may have particular advantages as an intervention in EDs and co-occurring mood or psychotic disorders. It can have efficacy even in low-weight patients who may not respond to medication due to the severity of their malnutrition and may provide an alternative for those who have unreasonable risk of medication side effects due to ED behaviors or who struggle to take medication. Although ECT can be a highly effective intervention, it is nevertheless a significant procedure that requires additional informed consent. Use of ECT in cases in which patients lack capacity varies from state to state and can include separate hearings, guardians, and other protective measures (Weiner 2003).

In patients with severe EDs, symptoms may be more amenable to change if mood or psychotic disorders are effectively treated. Considering ECT in patients with severe EDs involves considering the risks of the procedure related to medical compromise due to eating-disordered behaviors as well as the risks inherent in ECT. The procedure involves general anesthesia and requires a period of nothing by mouth prior. ECT may exacerbate risks related to the impaired cardiovascular function associated with EDs, including electrolyte abnormalities, cardiomyopathy, bradycardia, hypotension, and QTc prolongation (Pullen et al. 2011). Anesthesia carries its own risks to patients with a severe ED, including impaired glucose control, leukocytopenia leading to increased risk of periprocedural infection, and hypothermia. Anesthetic agents should be dosed according to obvious body weight and with consideration of the potential for myopathy related to weight suppression that may impact recovery from neuromuscular blockade (Hirose et al. 2014). ECT should be performed by practitioners who have experience treating patients with severe EDs, and the patients' current medical status should be carefully evaluated prior to each treatment, including their current ED behaviors. ECT should not be performed during times of acute refeeding, pulmonary compromise, or acute medical instability (Hirose et al. 2014; Saito 2005). The ability to adequately contain eating-disordered behaviors in the periods between ECT treatments and to support nutritional needs despite periods of interruption should be considered when undertaking ECT in patients with SEEDs. Although no large-scale studies for ECT in the treatment of EDs have been published, there are case reports of diverse patients who have successfully responded to this intervention, including adolescent patients, geriatric patients, and a case of a male with severe obesity and BED, likely due to adequately addressing co-occurring mood or psychotic disorders (Andrews et al. 2014; Hill et al. 2001; Rapinesi et al. 2013a, 2013b).

Neurofeedback

Neurofeedback is the voluntary regulation of brain activity in response to real-time information about brain activity from electroencephalography or functional MRI. Using software, individuals are presented either with a visual representation of their electroencephalographic data or changes in cerebral blood flow in specific patterns or with a game or task controlled by electroencephalography or functional MRI data. Participants are instructed to find a mental process that allows them to be successful in altering their electroencephalogram or cerebral blood flow or to complete the game or task (Collura 2000). Programs are designed to influence the production of different brainwaves or parts of the brain that, in turn, influence one's experience. The desired outcome will help determine where and how many electrodes should be placed in electroencephalography-supported neurofeedback and how many sessions should be undertaken, ranging from 1 to 6 or more sites and 1 to 100 or more sessions (Barreiros et al. 2019; Marzbani et al. 2016). In 22 adolescent females with AN, an electroencephalographic neurofeedback protocol targeted alpha frequencies, which are associated with awake relaxed states. In this study, reported restriction and dieting decreased and disinhibition increased; improvements in emotion regulation and emotion identification following engagement in neurofeedback were also found (Lackner et al. 2016). Neurofeedback has also been used to target overeating and disinhibited eating in patients with subclinical BED, which resulted in a decrease in overeating episodes and overvaluation of food (Ihssen et al. 2017; Schmidt and Martin 2015).

Virtual Reality Therapy

Virtual reality is "a three-dimensional, computer-generated environment [in which a] person becomes part of this virtual world or is immersed within this environment" (Virtual Reality Society 2017). Using technology, the person's sensory experience is modified to create an illusion that can feel real. Virtual reality therapy has been used successfully in anxiety disorders, phobias, PTSD, and schizophrenia (Maples-Keller et al. 2017). It has been used in the assessment of EDs using virtual food environments and as a therapeutic tool to address body image distortions and create exposures to challenging environments, such as a kitchen or scale. Following treatment, which ranged from a single intervention to several sessions per week for up to 8 weeks, and with follow-up data up to 1 year posttreatment, patients who received the virtual reality interventions demonstrated improvements in body attitudes, eating behaviors, and, in the case of patients with obesity and binge eating, weight loss (Cesa et al. 2013; de Carvalho et al. 2017).

Novel Psychotherapies

Psychotherapeutic interventions for severe EDs have been complicated by psychological and neurobiological factors specific to SEEDs. Patients often present with ambivalence to change or resistance to giving up the ED, anosognosia, difficulty recognizing that they have such a severe ED, and brain changes due to starvation during critical neurodevelopmental phases that can impact their ability to engage in psychotherapy (Treasure and Russell 2011; Vandereycken 2006). Nevertheless, psychological factors may be an important component in the maintenance of severe EDs, including cognitive rigidity, avoidance, obsessionality, and perfectionism (Latzer and Stein 2019). These factors may provide novel targets for which new psychotherapies can be tailored.

Family therapy is a well-proven intervention for adolescents and young adults with EDs, and women in recovery from EDs have identified supportive partners as an important component of their recovery (Fisher et al. 2018; Tozzi et al. 2003). Uniting Couples (in the treatment of) Anorexia Nervosa integrates cognitive-behavioral therapy for AN and couples therapy with individual therapy and medical interventions. Couples-based interventions include building skills such as communication and problem solving as well as positive interactions between partners. Supporting both members of a partnership during the treatment of an ED allows opportunities to interrupt inadvertent enabling behaviors that may perpetuate the disorder while strengthening the partnership against the disorder and increasing relationship satisfaction (Bulik et al. 2011; Kirby et al. 2016).

Cognitive inflexibility has been associated with EDs and persists beyond weight restoration (Roberts et al. 2007). Cognitive remediation therapy addresses these specific cognitive styles by introducing seemingly simple tasks that target cognitive processes using working memory, planning, and flexibility. In patients with AN, this therapy has evidence to support improvements in neurocognitive targets (Lindvall Dahlgren and Rø 2014).

Exposure and response prevention (ERP) therapy has traditionally been used in the treatment of OCD. ERP for AN targets specific food or eating anxieties and avoidance behaviors by creating exposures to feared situations and encouraging patients to not avoid their fear, creating habituation to the feared food item or experience and decreasing anxiety. It has supported increased caloric intake and decreased food-avoidant behaviors in patients with AN, but patients specifically with SEEDs have not been targeted (Farrell et al. 2019; Steinglass et al. 2012). In a patient population with SEEDs, it is important to consider the brain's ability to habituate to anxiety stimuli without nutritional rehabilitation.

Specialist-supportive clinical management is a therapeutic approach for AN that combines clinical management with supportive psychotherapy. It targets clinical goals and uses supportive psychotherapy to support change. In appointments, patients identify and target eating-disordered behaviors. A supportive psychotherapeutic stance includes providing support, acceptance, affection, and hope while respecting patients' defenses, focusing on their strengths, and helping them realize their ability to achieve goals independently. This intervention has been evaluated only in outpatients and, in trials, has shown efficacy consistent with cognitive-behavioral therapy, but it has been associated with high dropout rates (McIntosh 2015; Robinson et al. 2016).

Maudsley Anorexia Nervosa Treatment for Adults uses psychotherapy to target factors related to maintenance of disease, including obsessional and anxious/avoidant personality traits (e.g., thinking style, socioemotional avoidance, pro-AN beliefs) and the response of support persons to the disease, including anxiety, blame, or hostility. Using motivational interviewing and collaborative case formulation focusing on strengths and use of support persons as necessary, this approach aims to support behavioral change. At 2 years, improvements in BMI and ED symptoms, decreases in clinical impairment, and limited need for higher levels of care were found in an outpatient population; however, thus far the intervention has been limited to outpatients and has excluded patients who required inpatient treatment for life-threatening concerns (Schmidt et al. 2013, 2016).

Animal Therapy

Animal-assisted therapy has been evaluated in severe mental illness and in the treatment of EDs. Limited literature supports positive outcomes from these interventions. Following intervention, patients rated improvements in self-efficacy and coping skills and reductions in ED symptoms (Berget et al. 2008; Cumella et al. 2014). Service animals are animals trained for a specific task to assist someone with a disability, which can include mental illness; are protected by the Americans with Disabilities Act; and are allowed to accompany their owners to perform their duties (Clay 2016). In many states, it is illegal to misrepresent an animal as a service animal, with consequences including fines and felony charges (Animal Legal and Historical Center 2019). Emotional support animals are a broad, somewhat undefined category of animals that provide emotional support to their owners. No literature exists discussing the objective experience of patients with EDs and the use of these support animals; however, many concerns are being raised about the animals' training and their ability to safely accompany their owners (Firozi 2019). Prescribing for an emotional support animal has unclear legal and ethical implications if the animal is aggressive, and more restrictions are being placed on such animals due to aggressive incidents (U.S. Department of Transportation 2019; Younggren et al. 2016).

Feeding and Dietary Interventions

Microbiota

The intestinal microbiota is a symbiotic community of microorganisms that live in the human gut. The gut microbiome of each person is unique and is influenced by numerous factors, including the person's diet, environment, genetics, medications, and general health. In turn, the microbiome influences energy homeostasis, disease, food tolerance, and mood and behavior (Thursby and Juge 2017). Furthermore, well-described changes occur in the gut microbiome following weight loss via dietary changes or surgical intervention (Seganfredo et al. 2017). Fecal samples from patients with AN have demonstrated significant microbial differences from those of age-matched control subjects (Morita et al. 2015). Clinical investigations are ongoing of both the use of gut microbiota to influence symptoms and the response of microbiota to nutritional treatment in patients with AN (BioGaia 2016; Ruusunen et al. 2019).

Type of Diet

The idea that changing one's diet may impact physical illness and mental health is not new, and patients with EDs are perhaps more vulnerable to this concept (Twilley and Graber 2018). Many patients with restrictive EDs believe that eliminating certain foods can result in improvement of their illness and often have attempted this intervention prior to seeking treatment. However, orthorexia and caloric restriction are inherently problematic. Gastric emptying is significantly delayed in patients with AN, with severity of malnutrition and duration of illness both associated with emptying abnormalities (Norris et al. 2016). Orthorexia and caloric restriction also often lead to bingeing, with or without compensatory behaviors (Goldschmidt et al. 2012; Koven and Abry 2015). Support currently exists for a more diverse meal plan, and normalizing the use of all food for nutrition can be a component of successful treatment (Schebendach et al. 2011).

Conclusion

The treatment of SEEDs is a complex and multifactorial undertaking. The development and use of novel treatments offers new avenues for symptom relief and recovery support when traditional methods have been unsuccessful. Innovative pharmacological therapies, neuromodulation and neurosurgery, psychotherapies, and complementary and alternative treatments offer a glimpse into the future of treatment options for patients impacted by the most severe EDs.

References

Accurso EC, Ciao AC, Fitzsimmons-Craft EE, et al: Is weight gain really a catalyst for broader recovery? The impact of weight gain on psychological symptoms in the treatment of adolescent anorexia nervosa. Behav Res Ther 56:1–6, 2014

Agabio R, Farci AMG, Curreli O, et al: Oxytocin nasal spray in the treatment of binge eating disorder and obesity: a pilot, randomized, double-blind trial. Clinical Pharmacology and Biopharmaceutics 5(2), 2016

Aigner M, Treasure J, Kaye W, et al: World Federation of Societies of Biological Psychiatry (WFSBP) guidelines for the pharmacological treatment of eating disorders. World J Biol Psychiatry 12(6):400–443, 2011

Andrews PJT, Seide M, Guarda AS, et al: Electroconvulsive therapy in an adolescent with severe major depression and anorexia nervosa. J Child Adolesc Psychopharmacol 24(2):94–98, 2014

Andries A, Frystyk J, Flyvbjerg A, et al: Dronabinol in severe, enduring anorexia nervosa: a randomized controlled trial. Int J Eat Disord 47(1):18–23, 2014

Animal Legal and Historical Center: Fraudulent Service Dogs. East Lansing, MI, 2019. Available at: https://www.animallaw.info/content/fraudulent-service-dogs. Accessed August 25, 2019.

Avraham Y, Latzer Y, Hasid D, Berry EM: The impact of delta9-THC on the psychological symptoms of anorexia nervosa: a pilot study. Isr J Psychiatry Relat Sci 54(3):44–51, 2017

Bajgoric S, Samra K, Chandrapalan S, Gautam N: Cannabinoid hyperemesis syndrome: a guide for the practising clinician. BMJ Case Rep 2015

Barreiros AR, Almeida I, Baía BC, Castelo-Branco M: Amygdala modulation during emotion regulation training with fMRI-based neurofeedback. Front Hum Neurosci 13:89, 2019

Berget B, Ekeberg Ø, Braastad BO: Animal-assisted therapy with farm animals for persons with psychiatric disorders: effects on self-efficacy, coping ability and quality of life, a randomized controlled trial. Clin Pract Epidemiol Ment Health 4(1):9, 2008

BioGaia AB: The Role of Lactobacillus Reuteri in Children and Adolescents With Anorexia Nervosa. ClinicalTrials.gov, 2016. Available at: https://clinicaltrials.gov/ct2/show/NCT02004288. Accessed March 31, 2019.

Bloch M, Ish-Shalom S, Greenman Y, et al: Dehydroepiandrosterone treatment effects on weight, bone density, bone metabolism and mood in women suffering from anorexia nervosa: a pilot study. Psychiatry Res 200(2–3):544–549, 2012

Brownley KA, Von Holle A, Hamer RM, et al: A double-blind, randomized pilot trial of chromium picolinate for binge eating disorder: results of the Binge Eating and Chromium (BEACh) Study. J Psychosom Res 75(1):36–42, 2013

Brunelin J, Mondino M, Bation R, et al: Transcranial direct current stimulation for obsessive-compulsive disorder: a systematic review. Brain Sci 8(2):37, 2018

Bulik CM, Baucom D, Kirby J, Pisetsky E: Uniting Couples (in the treatment of Anorexia Nervosa (UCAN). Int J Eat Disord 44(1):19–28, 2011

Cesa GL, Manzoni GM, Bacchetta M, et al: Virtual reality for enhancing the cognitive behavioral treatment of obesity with binge eating disorder: randomized controlled study with one-year follow-up. J Med Internet Res 15(6), 2013

Clay RA: Is that a pet or therapeutic aid? Monitor on Psychology 47(8):38, 2016

Collura TF: Practical Issues Concerning EEG Biofeedback Devices, Protocols and Methods (online), 2000. Available at: http://openeeg.sourceforge.net/arch/att-0944/01-part. Accessed August 19, 2019.

Cumella EJ, Lutter CB, Osborne AS, Kally Z: Equine therapy in the treatment of female eating disorder. SOP Transactions on Psychology 1(1):13–21, 2014

Dalton B, Campbell IC, Schmidt U: Neuromodulation and neurofeedback treatments in eating disorders and obesity. Curr Opin Psychiatry 30(6):458–473, 2017

Dalton B, Bartholdy S, Campbell IC, Schmidt U: Neurostimulation in clinical and sub-clinical eating disorders: a systematic update of the literature. Curr Neuropharmacol 16(8):1174–1192, 2018a

Dalton B, Bartholdy S, McClelland J, et al: Randomised controlled feasibility trial of real versus sham repetitive transcranial magnetic stimulation treatment in adults with severe and enduring anorexia nervosa: The TIARA study. BMJ Open, 8(7), 2018b

de Carvalho MR, Dias TRS, Duchesne M, et al: Virtual reality as a promising strategy in the assessment and treatment of bulimia nervosa and binge eating disorder: a systematic review. Behav Sci (Basel) 7(3):43, 2017

Devlin MJ, Kissileff HR, Zimmerli EJ, et al: Gastric emptying and symptoms of bulimia nervosa: effect of a prokinetic agent. Physiol Behav 106(2):238–242, 2012

Downar J, Sankar A, Giacobbe P, et al: Unanticipated rapid remission of refractory bulimia nervosa, during high-dose repetitive transcranial magnetic stimulation of the dorsomedial prefrontal cortex: a case report. Front Psychiatry 3:30, 2012

Farrell NR, Bowie OR, Cimperman MM, et al: Exploring the preliminary effectiveness and acceptability of food-based exposure therapy for eating disorders: a case series of adult inpatients. J Exp Psychopathol 10(1):1–9, 2019

Fazeli PK, Lawson EA, Faje AT, et al: Treatment with a ghrelin agonist in outpatient women with anorexia nervosa: a randomized clinical trial. J Clin Psychiatry 79(1), 2018

Firozi P: An "emotional-support dog" attacked him on a flight. He's suing Delta and the owner. The Washington Post, May 29, 2019. Available at: https://www.washingtonpost.com/transportation/2019/05/29/an-emotional-support-dog-attacked-him-flight-hes-suing-delta-owner. Accessed August 25, 2019.

Fisher CA, Skocic S, Rutherford KA, Hetrick SE: Family therapy approaches for anorexia nervosa. Cochrane Database Syst Rev (10):CD004780, 2018

Forcano L, Mata F, de la Torre R, Verdejo-Garcia A: Cognitive and neuromodulation strategies for unhealthy eating and obesity: systematic review and discussion of neurocognitive mechanisms. Neurosci Biobehav Rev 87:161–191, 2018

Goldschmidt AB, Wall M, Loth KA, et al: Which dieters are at risk for the onset of binge-eating? A prospective study of adolescents and young adults. J Adolesc Health 51(1):86–92, 2012

Guerdjikova AI, Walsh B, Shan K, et al: Concurrent improvement in both binge eating and depressive symptoms with naltrexone/bupropion therapy in overweight or obese subjects with major depressive disorder in an open-label, uncontrolled study. Adv Ther 34(10):2307–2315, 2017

Guerdjikova AI, Williams S, Blom TJ, et al: Combination phentermine-topiramate extended release for the treatment of binge eating disorder: an open-label, prospective study. Innov Clin Neurosci 15(5–6):17–21, 2018

Hetman I, Brunstein Klomek A, Goldzweig G, et al: Percentage from target weight (PFTW) predicts re-hospitalization in adolescent anorexia nervosa. Isr J Psychiatry Relat Sci 54(3):28–34, 2017

Hill R, Haslett C, Kumar S: Anorexia nervosa in an elderly woman. Aust NZ J Psychiatry 35(2):246–248, 2001

Hirose K, Hirose M, Tanaka K, et al: Perioperative management of severe anorexia nervosa. Br J Anaesth 112(2):246–254, 2014

Horowitz S: Transcranial magnetic stimulation and cranial electrotherapy stimulation: treatments for psychiatric and neurologic disorders. Altern Complement Ther 19(4):188–193, 2013

Ihssen N, Sokunbi MO, Lawrence AD, et al: Neurofeedback of visual food cue reactivity: a potential avenue to alter incentive sensitization and craving. Brain Imaging Behav 11(3):915–924, 2017

Imbert S, Rat P, de Beaurepaire R: Baclofen treatment of bulimia nervosa and binge eating disorder: an internet survey. Ann Nutr Disord Ther 4(3), 2017

Israely M, Ram A, McCulloch Brandeis R, et al: A double blind, randomized crossover trial of tyrosine treatment on cognitive function and psychological parameters in severe hospitalized anorexia nervosa patients. Isr J Psychiatry Relat Sci 54(3):52–58, 2017

Järvinen A, Laine MK, Tikkanen R, Castrén ML: Beneficial effects of GLP-1 agonist in a male with compulsive food-related behavior associated with autism. Front Psychiatry 10:97, 2019

Johnson JW, Kotermanski SE: Mechanism of action of memantine. Curr Opin Pharmacol 6(1):61–67, 2006

Kekic M, McClelland J, Bartholdy S, et al: Single-session transcranial direct current stimulation temporarily improves symptoms, mood, and self-regulatory control in bulimia nervosa: a randomised controlled trial. PLoS ONE 12(1):e0167606, 2017

Kim S-H, Chung J-H, Kim T-H, et al: The effects of repetitive transcranial magnetic stimulation on eating behaviors and body weight in obesity: a randomized controlled study. Brain Stimul 11(3):528–535, 2018

Kim Y-R, Kim C-H, Cardi V, et al: Intranasal oxytocin attenuates attentional bias for eating and fat shape stimuli in patients with anorexia nervosa. Psychoneuroendocrinology 44:133–142, 2014

Kirby JS, Fischer MS, Raney TJ, et al: Couple-based interventions in the treatment of adult anorexia nervosa: a brief case example of UCAN. Psychotherapy (Chic) 53(2):241–250, 2016

Knyahnytska YO, Blumberger DM, Daskalakis ZJ, et al: Insula H-coil deep transcranial magnetic stimulation in severe and enduring anorexia nervosa (SE-AN): a pilot study. Neuropsychiatr Dis Treat 15:2247–2256, 2019

Koven NS, Abry AW: The clinical basis of orthorexia nervosa: emerging perspectives. Neuropsychiatr Dis Treat 11:385–394, 2015

Lackner N, Unterrainer H-F, Skliris D, et al: EEG neurofeedback effects in the treatment of adolescent anorexia nervosa. Eat Disord 24(4):354–374, 2016

Lafrance A, Loizaga-Velder A, Fletcher J, et al: Nourishing the spirit: exploratory research on ayahuasca experiences along the continuum of recovery from eating disorders. J Psychoactive Drugs 49(5):427–435, 2017

Latzer Y, Stein D: Introduction: Novel perspectives on the psychology and psychotherapy of eating disorders. J Clin Psychol 75(8):1369–1379, 2019

Leroy A, Carton L, Gomajee H, et al: Naltrexone in the treatment of binge eating disorder in a patient with severe alcohol use disorder: a case report. Am J Drug Alcohol Abuse 43(5):618–620, 2017

Lindvall Dahlgren C, Rø Ø: A systematic review of cognitive remediation therapy for anorexia nervosa: development, current state and implications for future research and clinical practice. J Eat Disord 2(1):26, 2014

Lipsman N, Woodside DB, Giacobbe P, Lozano AM: Neurosurgical treatment of anorexia nervosa: review of the literature from leucotomy to deep brain stimulation. Eur Eat Disord Rev 21(6):428–435, 2013

Lipsman N, Lam E, Volpini M, et al: Deep brain stimulation of the subcallosal cingulate for treatment-refractory anorexia nervosa: 1 year follow-up of an open-label trial. Lancet Psychiatry 4(4):285–294, 2017

Lozano AM, Lipsman N, Bergman H, et al: Deep brain stimulation: current challenges and future directions. Nat Rev Neurol 15(3):148–160, 2019

Maples-Keller JL, Bunnell BE, Kim S-J, Rothbaum BO: The use of virtual reality technology in the treatment of anxiety and other psychiatric disorders. Harv Rev Psychiatry 25(3):103–113, 2017

Maranhão MF, Estella NM, Cury MEG, et al: The effects of repetitive transcranial magnetic stimulation in obese females with binge eating disorder: a protocol for a double-blinded, randomized, sham-controlled trial. BMC Psychiatry 15(1):194, 2015

Marazziti D, Piccinni A, Baroni S, Dell'Osso L: Effectiveness of nalmefene in binge eating disorder: a case report. J Clin Psychopharmacol 36(1):103–104, 2016

Marzbani H, Marateb HR, Mansourian M: Neurofeedback: a comprehensive review on system design, methodology and clinical applications. Basic Clin Neurosci 7(2):143–158, 2016

Mauri M, Miniati M, Mariani MG, et al: Haloperidol for severe anorexia nervosa restricting type with delusional body image disturbance: a nine-case chart review. Eat Weight Disord 18(3):329–332, 2013

McElroy SL, Guerdjikova AI, Winstanley EL, et al: Sodium oxybate in the treatment of binge eating disorder: an open-label, prospective study. Int J Eat Disord 44(3):262–268, 2011

McElroy SL, Guerdjikova AI, Mori N, et al: Armodafinil in binge eating disorder: a randomized, placebo-controlled trial. Int Clin Psychopharmacol 30(4):209–215, 2015a

McElroy SL, Guerdjikova AI, Mori N, et al: Psychopharmacologic treatment of eating disorders: emerging findings. Curr Psychiatry Rep 17(5):35, 2015b

McIntosh V: Specialist supportive clinical management (SSCM) for anorexia nervosa: content analysis, change over course of therapy, and relation to outcome. J Eat Disord 3(S1):O1, 2015

Mills IH, Park GR, Manara AR, Merriman RJ: Treatment of compulsive behaviour in eating disorders with intermittent ketamine infusions. QJM 91(7):493–503, 1998

Misra M, Katzman DK, Estella NM, et al: Impact of physiologic estrogen replacement on anxiety symptoms, body shape perception, and eating attitudes in adolescent girls with anorexia nervosa: data from a randomized controlled trial. J Clin Psychiatry 74(8):e765–e771, 2013

Morita C, Tsuji H, Hata T, et al: Gut dysbiosis in patients with anorexia nervosa. PLoS One 10(12):e0145274, 2015

Mustonen A, Niemelä S, Nordström T, et al: Adolescent cannabis use, baseline prodromal symptoms and the risk of psychosis. Br J Psychiatry 212(4):227–233, 2018

Norris ML, Harrison ME, Isserlin L, et al: Gastrointestinal complications associated with anorexia nervosa: a systematic review. Int J Eat Disord 49(3):216–237, 2016

Park RJ, Scaife JC, Aziz TZ: Study protocol: using deep brain stimulation, multimodal neuroimaging and neuroethics to understand and treat severe enduring anorexia nervosa. Front Psychiatry 9:24, 2018

Pattathan MB, Hejazi RA, McCallum RW: Association of marijuana use and cyclic vomiting syndrome. Pharmaceuticals 5(7):719, 2012

Popik P, Kos T, Zhang Y, Bisaga A: Memantine reduces consumption of highly palatable food in a rat model of binge eating. Amino Acids 40(2):477–485, 2011

Prinz P, Stengel A: Deep brain stimulation: possible treatment strategy for pathologically altered body weight? Brain Sci 8(1):19, 2018

Pullen SJ, Rasmussen KG, Angstman ER, et al: The safety of electroconvulsive therapy in patients with prolonged QTc intervals on the electrocardiogram. J ECT 27(3):192–200, 2011

Rapinesi C, Del Casale A, Serata D, et al: Electroconvulsive therapy in a man with comorbid severe obesity, binge eating disorder, and bipolar disorder. J ECT 29(2):142–144, 2013a

Rapinesi C, Serata D, Del Casale A, et al: Effectiveness of electroconvulsive therapy in a patient with a treatment-resistant major depressive episode and comorbid body dysmorphic disorder. J ECT 29(2):145–146, 2013b

Ricoux O, Carton L, Ménard O, et al: Acute psychosis related to baclofen in a patient treated for binge eating disorder highlights the urgent need to regulate off-label prescriptions. J Clin Psychopharmacol 39(3):282–284, 2019

Roberts ME, Tchanturia K, Stahl D, et al: A systematic review and meta-analysis of set-shifting ability in eating disorders. Psychol Med 37(8):1075–1084, 2007

Robinson P, Hellier J, Barrett B, et al: The NOURISHED randomised controlled trial comparing mentalisation-based treatment for eating disorders (MBT-ED) with specialist supportive clinical management (SSCM-ED) for patients with eating disorders and symptoms of borderline personality disorder. Trials 17(1):549, 2016

Rotroff DM, Corum DG, Motsinger-Reif A, et al: Metabolomic signatures of drug response phenotypes for ketamine and esketamine in subjects with refractory major depressive disorder: new mechanistic insights for rapid acting antidepressants. Transl Psychiatry 6(9):e894, 2016

Russell J, Maguire S, Hunt GE, et al: Intranasal oxytocin in the treatment of anorexia nervosa: randomized controlled trial during re-feeding. Psychoneuroendocrinology 87:83–92, 2018

Ruusunen A, Rocks T, Jacka F, Loughman A: The gut microbiome in anorexia nervosa: relevance for nutritional rehabilitation. Psychopharmacology 236(5):1545–1558, 2019

Saito S: Anesthesia management for electroconvulsive therapy: hemodynamic and respiratory management. J Anesth 19(2):142–149, 2005

Salik I, Marwaha R: Electroconvulsive therapy, in StatPearls. Tampa, FL, StatPearls Publishing, 2019. Available at: https://www.ncbi.nlm.nih.gov/books/NBK538266. Accessed March 31, 2019.

Schebendach JE, Mayer LE, Devlin MJ, et al: Food choice and diet variety in weight-restored patients with anorexia nervosa. J Am Diet Assoc 111(5):732–736, 2011

Schmidt J, Martin A: Neurofeedback reduces overeating episodes in female restrained eaters: a randomized controlled pilot-study. Appl Psychophysiol Biofeedback 40(4):283–295, 2015

Schmidt U, Renwick B, Lose A, et al: The MOSAIC study: comparison of the Maudsley Model of Treatment for Adults with Anorexia Nervosa (MANTRA) with Specialist Supportive Clinical Management (SSCM) in outpatients with anorexia nervosa or eating disorder not otherwise specified, anorexia nervosa type: study protocol for a randomized controlled trial. Trials 14:160, 2013

Schmidt U, Ryan EG, Bartholdy S, et al: Two-year follow-up of the MOSAIC trial: a multicenter randomized controlled trial comparing two psychological treatments in adult outpatients with broadly defined anorexia nervosa. Int J Eat Disord 49(8):793–800, 2016

Seganfredo FB, Blume CA, Moehlecke M, et al: Weight-loss interventions and gut microbiota changes in overweight and obese patients: a systematic review: weight-loss impact on gut microbiota. Obes Rev 18(8):832–851, 2017

Steinglass J, Albano AM, Simpson HB, et al: Fear of food as a treatment target: exposure and response prevention for anorexia nervosa in an open series. Int J Eat Disord 45(4):615–621, 2012

Steinglass J, Kaplan SC, Liu Y, et al: The (lack of) effect of alprazolam on eating behavior in anorexia nervosa: a preliminary report. Int J Eat Disord 47(8):901–904, 2014

Thair H, Holloway AL, Newport R, Smith AD: Transcranial direct current stimulation (tDCS): a beginner's guide for design and implementation. Front Neurosci 11:641, 2017

Thomas G, Lucas P, Capler N, et al: Ayahuasca-assisted therapy for addiction: results from a preliminary observational study in Canada. Curr Drug Abuse Rev 6(1):30–42, 2013

Thursby E, Juge N: Introduction to the human gut microbiota. Biochem J 474(11):1823–1836, 2017

Touyz S, Hay P: Severe and enduring anorexia nervosa (SE-AN): in search of a new paradigm. J Eat Disord 3(1):26, 2015

Touyz S, Le Grange D, Lacey H, et al: Treating severe and enduring anorexia nervosa: a randomized controlled trial. Psychol Med 43(12):2501–2511, 2013

Tozzi F, Sullivan PF, Fear JL, et al: Causes and recovery in anorexia nervosa: the patient's perspective. Int J Eat Disord 33(2):143–154, 2003

Treasure J, Russell G: The case for early intervention in anorexia nervosa: theoretical exploration of maintaining factors. Br J Psychiatry 199(1):5–7, 2011

Twilley N, Graber C: The ancient origins of dieting. The Atlantic, January 30, 2018. Available at https://www.theatlantic.com/health/archive/2018/01/the-ancient-origins-of-dieting/551828. Accessed April 5, 2019.

U.S. Department of Transportation: Final statement of enforcement priorities regarding service animals, August 8, 2019. Available at: https://www.transportation.gov/individuals/aviation-consumer-protection/final-statement-enforcement-priorities-service-animals. Accessed August 25, 2019.

U.S. Drug Enforcement Administration: Drug Scheduling (online), 2019. Available at: https://www.dea.gov/drug-scheduling. Accessed August 22, 2019.

Van den Eynde F, Guillaume S, Broadbent H, et al: Repetitive transcranial magnetic stimulation in anorexia nervosa: a pilot study. Eur Psychiatry 28(2):98–101, 2013

Vandereycken W: Denial of illness in anorexia nervosa: a conceptual review. Part 2: different forms and meanings. Eur Eat Disord Rev 14(5):352–368, 2006

Virtual Reality Society: What is Virtual Reality (online)? 2017. Available at: https://www.vrs.org.uk/virtual-reality/what-is-virtual-reality.html. Accessed March 29, 2019.

Volkow ND, Swanson JM, Evins AE, et al: Effects of cannabis use on human behavior, including cognition, motivation, and psychosis: a review. JAMA Psychiatry 73(3):292–297, 2016

Walpoth M, Hoertnagl C, Mangweth-Matzek B, et al: Repetitive transcranial magnetic stimulation in bulimia nervosa: preliminary results of a single-centre, randomised, double-blind, sham-controlled trial in female outpatients. Psychother Psychosom 77(1):57–60, 2008

Weiner RD: Ethical considerations with electroconvulsive therapy. AMA J Ethics 5(10):352–354, 2003

Westmoreland P, Krantz MJ, Mehler PS: Medical complications of anorexia nervosa and bulimia nervosa. Am J Med 129(1):30–37, 2016

Whiting DM, Tomycz ND, Bailes J, et al: Lateral hypothalamic area deep brain stimulation for refractory obesity: a pilot study with preliminary data on safety, body weight, and energy metabolism. J Neurosurg 119(1):56–63, 2013

Woodside DB, Colton P, Lam E, et al: Dorsomedial prefrontal cortex repetitive transcranial magnetic stimulation treatment of posttraumatic stress disorder in eating disorders: an open-label case series. Int J Eat Disord 50(10):1231–1234, 2017

Yager J, Devlin MJ, Halmi K, et al: Practice Guidelines for the Treatment of Patients With Eating Disorders, 3rd Edition. Arlington, VA, American Psychiatric Association, 2010

Younggren JN, Boisvert JA, Boness CL: Examining emotional support animals and role conflicts in professional psychology. Prof Psychol Res Pract 47(4):255–260, 2016

9

Harm Reduction

Ovidio Bermudez, M.D., FAAP, FSAHM, FAED, Fiaedp, C.E.D.S.
Phillipa Hay, M.D.
Stephen Touyz, Ph.D.

THE concept that human disease causes harm in both the short and long term is not new. Ideally, we would prevent disease or treat it with the goal of avoiding harm altogether. The public health literature refers to interventions that prevent problems or diseases from emerging as *primary* or *universal* preventions, such as immunizations. When prevention is not attainable, the next best options are interventions to reverse or preclude harm from exposure to known risk factors. Addressing a given illness as early as possible to prevent sequelae is known as *secondary* or *targeted* prevention. The last option, *tertiary* prevention (Caplan 1964), is to implement interventions to reduce rather than reverse harm in the most severely impacted individuals. The aim of this intervention is to prevent the severe negative effects of an enduring illness or condition, with the goal not only of preserving a life but also of improving the quality of that life.

In some instances, avoiding harm caused by an illness is neither possible nor realistic. Harm is inevitable. At such times, the focus can shift to mitigating the degree of harm and its impact on quality of life, referred to as a *harm reduction model* of disease management or *harm minimization*. Implicit in this term is that the goal is not to eradicate the disease or prevent all harm but to reduce the damage it causes and improve the life experiences and the quality of life opportunities for individuals with the underlying illness. The decision to embark on harm reduction does not need to be irreversible; the door remains open either to taking further steps in greater harm reduction or to curing or eradicating the illness as treatments advance or patients' acceptance of and tolerability to treatment allow.

In this chapter, we explore a harm reduction model of disease management for eating disorders (EDs). This poses two practical and ethical challenges. First, the consensus on defining "recovery" from an ED is limited (Khalsa et al. 2017). Second, the definition of *chronicity* in a group of serious mental illnesses (e.g., anorexia nervosa [AN] and bulimia nervosa]) must consider that due to the early age at onset (adolescence) and because the opportunity for recovery for many falls within a 7- to 10-year period that often coincides with full brain maturation (mid- to late twenties), patients who have been ill for several years should not necessarily be labeled "chronic" or "not responsive to treatment efforts." Recent literature illustrates the notion that some patients do have hope of improvement or recovery, even after having an ED for 20 years or longer (Eddy et al. 2017). Often, this is when patients reach a "tipping point" frequently described by people who recover (Dawson et al. 2014; Hay et al. 2013). In addition, in AN in particular, we are dealing with the added complexity of an ego-syntonic stance toward the illness for most patients, especially in the early course of the illness, when patients who might otherwise respond positively to treatment prefer to limit their weight and nutritional recovery due to intolerance of weight gain or food intake. When this occurs, not only do they diminish their chances for a positive early response to treatment but they also may derail brain development, which is one of the best opportunities for strong and lasting recovery when onset occurs in the teen years. When considering a harm reduction model, one approach is to view these patients as meeting criteria for severe and enduring eating disorder (SEED) or severe and enduring anorexia nervosa (SEAN). Of interest, the concept of "severe and enduring" in psychiatry was coined in 1999 as "severe and enduring mental illness" in a publication from the U.K. Department of Health entitled *National Service Framework for Mental Health* (Robinson 2014).

We propose that in AN, many but not all patients may experience three phases: enamored, ambivalent, and disillusioned. This should be kept in mind when assessing a patient who requests a harm reduction approach. Harm reduction can also be viewed as a step before palliative/hospice care or reaching a conclusion of treatment futility. These patients often find resistance to continued treatment support in both single- and multiple-party payment systems (Kaplan and Buchanan 2012; Lopez et al. 2010). Given these added financial barriers to treatment and the inability to effect behavior change in the patient, it is possible one may reach the conclusion of treatment unresponsiveness or treatment futility prematurely.

Another layer of complexity is the lack of evidence-based approaches to treat SEED/SEAN (Hay et al. 2014; Touyz et al. 2013). The definition of what constitutes "severe and enduring" is still evolving; in 2013, Stephen

Touyz and colleagues made the case for a different paradigm to treatment as usual for this subset of patients with the most severe forms of eating pathology. They called for treatment efforts to "focus on retention, improved quality of life with harm minimization, and avoidance of further failure experiences." In their study, adult patients with SEAN (>7 years of symptoms) randomized to receive either cognitive-behavioral therapy (CBT) for AN or specialist-supported clinical management had improved equally at the end of treatment. However, at follow-up, those who received CBT showed statistically significant benefits. At 6 months, they had higher scores on the Weismann Social Adjustment Scale (Weissman and Bothwell 1976), and at 12-month follow-up, they had lower scores on the Eating Disorders Examination (Fairburn and Cooper 1993) and higher readiness for recovery. This highlights that another aspect of defining SEED or SEAN may be to assess whether individuals with longstanding symptoms have received adequate and evidence-based treatment efforts and how to best define those. Number and quality of past treatment efforts should also be considered (Broomfield et al. 2017).

Harm reduction efforts should be driven by the desire to individualize care, recognize and respect self-determination in competent patients, and meet patients where they are in their perception of their illness and desire or readiness for change (Table 9–1).

Practical Examples of Harm Reduction Approaches

At a practical level, either the patient or clinical team may propose a harm reduction approach. When it is proposed by a patient, deliberation should include the patient's motivation and degree of emotional or phobic threshold avoidance, the degree to which the patient's request for acceptance of some symptoms (versus *endorsement* of symptoms) by the clinical team is reasonable, and whether the plan will indeed be likely to reduce harm and improve the patient's quality of life. When proposed by a clinical team, it should include the factors discussed in the following sections.

Weight Expectation Reduction

When a patient with SEED fails to sustain a normal weight, the clinical team may agree to a lower target to reduce medical risk and improve quality of life. For example, for a patient who has maintained 60% of expected body weight (EBW) but been unable to sustain a weight above that or gained weight while in a 24-hour care setting only to lose it in a less restrictive setting, the team and patient may agree to set 85% of EBW as the harm reduction target for

TABLE 9–1.   What harm reduction in eating disorders is and is not

What harm reduction is:

A pragmatic personalized approach targeting reduction in negative consequences of risk behaviors.

A shift in the way an individual clinician or group of clinicians conceptualizes a case in which they are willing to prioritize extending life and preserving or improving quality of life for individuals with a severe and enduring eating disorder.

A step in the direction of considering alternatives to treatment without prioritizing (or excluding) the expectation of recovery or cure.

A step to be considered before palliative/hospice care or a conclusion of futility (Westmoreland and Mehler 2016) for a given patient who has received adequate and sufficient conventional treatment efforts.

What harm reduction is not:

A universal approach to eradicating risk behaviors.

An accommodation to individuals' treatment tolerance early in the course of their eating disorder or before they have had an opportunity to achieve weight normalization, nutritional rehabilitation, and interruption of compensatory behaviors.

A way for patients to practice emotional avoidance or avoidance of their fear threshold, for example, avoiding reaching their fear of weight.

A way for patients who are enamored with and willing to defend their illness to remain ill.

An ethical approach for minors or those with recent onset or treatment-naive eating disorders.

---

a specified period or indefinitely. If the patient can maintain this new weight goal, the target may be further advanced at a later time or be maintained for a longer period to reassess the feasibility of further improvements. If the patient is not able to maintain the new weight target (it may take more than one attempt), then he or she has not responded to a harm reduction model. The patient may argue that the target weight was set too high and that 80% is more sustainable, which may or may not be true; at this juncture, the clinical reasonableness of further reducing the weight target should be considered. At 80% EBW this patient may still reap some benefit of reduced medical risk and improved quality of life, but this is unlikely to be true at 70% EBW.

Purging Symptoms Reduction

Patients whose SEED includes persistent purging behaviors that put them at risk of severe medical complications or threatens their survival may be candidates for a harm reduction model targeting a reduction in the mode, frequency, or severity of these behaviors. Harm reduction expectations for a patient who is severely underweight and engaging in high levels of laxative abuse might include improving weight and diminishing the quantity and frequency of laxative use or modifying the type of laxative to a less harmful form. For example, a patient who has been at 70% EBW and using 100 tablets of stimulant laxatives daily may agree to bring her weight to 85% EBW and adhere to an agreed regimen of nonstimulant bowel aids. This regimen may be more than usually prescribed but much less harmful than excessive amounts of stimulant laxatives. Success would then be defined as maintaining a weight that is lower than normal but less severely underweight and abstaining from a high probability of medical issues caused by severe stimulant laxative abuse. A less desirable outcome would be the patient remaining at a very low weight, experiencing weight fluctuations related to relapse of stimulant laxative abuse, or continuing to abuse stimulant laxatives.

When considering a harm reduction model, the treatment team should also contemplate the possible consequences of this approach. For example, the lower a person's BMI and more fragile his or her physique, the higher the risk the person will develop an unrelated infectious illness or suffer the consequences of osteoporosis (e.g., sustaining vertebral fractures and becoming bedridden). Alternatively (or in addition), people who continue to use laxatives—albeit perhaps less frequently—may still end up with permanent damage to their colons, and patients who purge or use diuretics may still end up with chronic renal failure, despite lessening their use of these modalities.

Parallels From Other Fields

In addition to the EDs, harm reduction is practiced in other areas of medicine, some of which use the term explicitly and others not at all. In oncology, a physician may debulk a tumor that has been refractory to curative efforts with the intent of improving a patient's life expectancy and quality while remaining aware that eradication of the tumor is not possible. In such an instance, the physician employs the *spirit* of harm reduction but may not necessarily name it. The goals are to extend life, prevent further complications, and improve quality of life in the time remaining for the individual. In the medical management of obesity, achieving and sustaining the loss of large amounts of weight has proven to be elusive for most patients. Thus, modest loss of approximately 5%–10% of body weight is often advocated as a way to reduce medical complications and their impact (e.g., improving insulin resistance or sleep apnea) and improve patients' longevity and quality of life (e.g., improved ambulation or decreased joint pain in lower extremities). For severely overweight patients, maintaining 90% of their body weight does not resolve the overweight/obesity state but does reduce the medical harm that the condition may cause. This is a harm reduction model and is often referred to as such.

Although the goal when treating psychiatric disorders such as depression is full remission of symptoms, when the depression becomes chronic, reducing its symptom severity or modifying its risk factors may become the target of intervention; thus, improvement in functionality to some degree becomes the goal even as depression persists. With regard to schizophrenia, alternatives to addressing the illness rather than aiming for its full cure or eradication are also explored more consistently.

Addiction psychiatry is another example in which harm reduction has been implemented. In the 1980s, Phillip Brickman proposed four models of helping and coping to treat addictive behaviors that matched interventional approaches (Brickman et al. 1982). First is the moral model, which tends to enhance the patient's guilt, shame, and feelings of stigma; relies on punishments such as incarceration; and has a goal of abstinence. Second is the disease model, which does not blame patients or attempt to coerce them into abstinence but rather focuses on factors beyond their control, such as family history and genetic vulnerability. This model sees addiction as a progressive disease with no known cure in which abstinence is the only way to halt progression. The third model is a spiritual model, which endorses the disease model but relies on social support and believes in a higher power to achieve abstinence. Fourth is the compensatory model, which sees addictive behavior as caused by biopsychosocial factors that vary among individuals. Treatment consists of teaching patients to cope better with these factors and craft goals according to their needs and capabilities and may include abstinence or moderation. Harm reduction fits into this fourth model; in this context, it can be defined as an approach that meets people where they are, rather than force a dichotomized notion of use or abstinence. A harm reduction model in which the intent is not even to modify the extent of use is a needle and syringe exchange program, which does not attempt to curtail use but to decrease the life-threatening risk of infectious disease transmission via needle sharing (Marlatt and Witkiewitz 2010). Several international organizations, such as the World Health Organization, now embrace the term *harm reduction* (Wodak 2009).

Harm reduction in psychiatry also includes interventions to reduce self-harmful behaviors and suicide risk. Psychiatric illness is heterogeneous and complex. Patients often experience psychiatric comorbidity, and clear delineation of single psychiatric symptoms complexes is the exception rather than the rule. Thus, harm reduction in psychiatry needs to be fluid and illness- and situation-specific rather than a blanket approach to reducing risk or complications in disease management. Safety planning for those who are struggling with personal safety and at risk of self-harmful behaviors and suicide is also a form of harm reduction in mental health.

Accommodating Distress in an Ego-Syntonic Illness

Drawing the line between respecting patients' right to self-determination and colluding with their illness or enabling them to perpetuate potentially life-threatening symptoms to alleviate dysphoria or bring short-term relief is not an easy endeavor for mental health professionals. Patients may take a help-rejecting stance, struggle with ambivalence, or express their desire to change but be incapable of initiating or sustaining such actions. It is in some ways easier when patients fabricate motivation in an effort to "be left alone" in their ego-syntonicity; it is more difficult when patients truly desire improvement but are unable to consistently engage in behavior change during times of distress. For the latter, clinicians must deal with "two truths" and handle the dialectical dilemma of shifting expectations and inconsistencies in behavior. Thus, recognizing patient accommodation of the illness rather than gradual engagement in change becomes one of the important tasks of working with individuals with SEEDs. When clinicians, hoping for risk reduction, are lured into agreements or arrangements with patients that do not materialize in meaningful (albeit at times gradual) changes in behaviors, they face the pitfall of enabling ongoing symptomatology without the benefit of reducing risk. Well-intentioned clinicians may sometimes face this dilemma, and a high level of awareness is the only way to avoid these pitfalls and manage countertransference (Strober 2004).

Rationale for a Harm Reduction Approach

One may have different expectations when considering a harm reduction approach for patients with SEEDs. Some patients may have reached maximum benefit from treatment efforts aimed at recovery and thus may benefit from a shift in expectations toward minimizing health risk for the remainder of their illness course. In other words, the hoped-for outcome is to prolong the person's life while improving the quality of that life. Alternatively, some patients view a harm reduction model as "drop-in resistance" from the clinical team that lets them initiate change in what they perceive as "small degrees" rather than contemplate larger degrees of change that have proven intolerable in the past. Some, perhaps many, of these patients in our clinical experience go on to make further improvement and even recover fully. In other words, they may reach that tipping point mentioned earlier and be able to tolerate treatment and make further progress. Fear of initiating big change may be what has kept them stuck in their illness, and smaller doses of change may be more tolerable. An analogy that is helpful for some patients is that of climbing a mountain by going from one rest station to the next rather than aiming for the summit. Although there has been some resistance to the paradigm shift in favor of harm reduction for some patients, given that an increasing number of patients with AN end up meeting criteria for SEED/SEAN, we need to explore alternative best practices (Bamford et al. 2015).

For Which Patients Should We Consider Harm Reduction?

Until recently, literature denoting criteria for the use of a harm reduction model in ED treatment was limited. After all, the term *severe and enduring eating disorder* first appeared in the literature in 2008 (Arkell and Robinson 2008). In 2018, Hay and Touyz proposed criteria for patient inclusion in SEED/SEAN research that included functional impairment, poor quality of life, persistence of symptoms with negative physiological consequences, overvaluation based on weight or shape and other ED cognitions, duration of illness lasting at least 3 years, engagement in at least two evidence-based treatment efforts, and conceptualization of illness, including the patient's health literacy about EDs and stage of change. These authors did not discuss the potential impact of psychiatric comorbidity and how this may impact the burden of disease. This is another area in which further research is necessary to better understand who may be a candidate for a harm reduction approach.

Ethical Considerations

A harm reduction approach must take several ethical issues into account in order to ensure clinicians understand the patient's needs at a given time and make clinical decisions that are clearly in that patient's best interest. Principles such as "first do no harm" and respecting the patient's right to self-determination (taking capacity for decision making into account) should be used as guides. The question of patients in a younger age group who meet criteria for SEEDs—if accurately identified before a protracted course of illness, thus opening the door to alternative approaches—has recently been raised in the literature and poses another layer of complexity in ethical considerations (Kaplan and Strober 2019).

Harm Reduction May Serve as a Stepping Stone

It is important to not lock patients into a harm reduction approach forever but to verbalize that it is a stepping stone to support them in moving toward improved health and quality of life. Although this may not apply in circumstances in which permanent dysfunction has occurred, such as a patient for whom ED complications have led to chronic renal failure and a need for ongoing dialysis, in other instances, improvement can occur even if full recovery from an acquired dysfunction may not be possible. An example is chronic laxative abuse, in which complete normalization of bowel function may not be possible but improvement and decreased need for bowel aids may be possible with interrupted or reduced laxative use.

In other instances, full recovery of an acquired dysfunction may be possible. The particular behavior may need to be fully interrupted. An example of this is cyclical edema secondary to diuretic abuse. The only way to interrupt the cycle of recurrent fluid retention is to fully interrupt the diuretic abuse. Clinicians should always aim for ongoing minimization of medical and psychiatric risk to the extent possible and tolerated by patients, but leaving the door open to further revisions is just as important.

Harm Reduction Does Not Always Work

Clinicians and patients participating in a harm reduction approach need to recognize when the approach has proven not to be helpful and should be abandoned. There should be both clarity and a reasonable degree of flexibility on the part of all stakeholders. For example, a lapse in a stipulated goal may not automatically mean the effort is futile; if the patient lapsed in his or her effort to limit the number of laxatives taken per day, this may be an opportunity to clarify expectations and continue the effort. However, if such lapses became recurrent or fit into a new pattern of abuse, then the validity of the harm reduction agreement would have to be reexamined. Continuing a harm reduction approach for a prolonged period of time without actually achieving tangible risk reduction is contraindicated.

Guiding Ethical Principles: Benevolence and Nonmaleficence

Given that the ethics of working with patients with SEED or SEAN are addressed elsewhere in this book, we do not dwell extensively on the topic. However, in a harm reduction approach, the ethical principles of beneficence and nonmaleficence must be considered at every stage of the process. It is imperative to not err on either extreme. A harm reduction approach for a patient with SEED or SEAN cannot be based on accommodating the patient's illness or for the convenience of the clinical team. Not being open to the potential short- or long-term benefits of a harm reduction model may close an important door for some patients, but implementing such a model too early, in the wrong context, or without achieving the intended benefits for the patient may do more harm than good. The ethics around the clinical management of SEED/SEAN are complicated and may at times require expert consultation or ethical guidance even for the most experienced clinician. To avoid clinical burnout, clinicians must manage countertransference and ensure that they manage these patients voluntarily and with full understanding of the burden to caregivers. Clinical practice guidelines for the treatment of EDs published by the Royal Australian and New Zealand College of Psychiatrists include a section and important guidance on the management of SEED and SEAN and point to the value of a harm reduction or modified treatment expectations approach (Hay et al. 2014).

SEED is one of the most challenging disorders in mental health care (Wonderlich et al. 2012). Further understanding what differentiates it from other eating pathologies and advances in tailored interventions is needed to prevent the morbidity, mortality, and human suffering associated with these most severe forms of EDs.

In a Patient's Own Words

Following is the testimonial of a 45-year-old woman with SEED/SEAN:

> To me, a harm reduction model of care is a lifesaving approach for those individuals with severe and enduring anorexia nervosa. I was first diagnosed and hospitalized with anorexia nervosa at the age of 16 years. Unfortunately, I also suffered from severe comorbid symptoms of anxiety, depression, and

OCD. At that time, I was a talented tennis player and had won several competitions at a state level. There was even talk at that time that I should compete at the international level. However, I unfortunately relapsed each time that I was discharged from hospital and had to be readmitted. I was unable to complete my school education, leaving school at the age of 17 years.

The years that followed were devastating for me, with little or no prospect of a career and ever-decreasing health as a result of my protracted emaciation and laxative abuse. I had little or no energy, felt both anxious and depressed with marked compulsive rituals and the added diagnosis of osteoporosis. I found it almost impossible to continue with my tennis career, and I then lost the one thing in my life that I was passionate about and gave me a sense of being worthwhile. My self-esteem was shattered beyond repair. My life became empty, with nothing to aspire toward other than preserving my thinness. Nothing else mattered now. I felt I had lost my sense of identity.

I had one treatment experience where I was admitted to treatment involuntarily and my weight was normalized. I felt this was forced upon me, and in spite of feeling better physically, my obsession with bowel function was magnified, and right after discharge I quickly relapsed into restriction and laxative abuse and lost the weight rapidly. What followed can only best be described as decades of misery and despair. I was faced with revolving-door admissions to hospital, with none conferring any longer-term benefit. Each time I would gain some weight, albeit not very much, but on discharge I would lose it all again. My mental anguish continued unabated. I would inevitably relapse in laxative abuse. My family often questioned how I could continue to survive and what was stopping me from getting better....I tried to explain to them that it wasn't that I didn't want to get better and to overcome this debilitating disease that was ruining my life and theirs, it was that I was too terrified to change. Any weight gain devastated me, and the thought of doing so was just too difficult to contemplate. The despair that would follow was unthinkable. It is not that I did not want to play tennis again or to have a relationship; I could not see as to how I could live at a higher weight. I was well and truly trapped inside this illness with no way out.

I also came to the conclusion that all eating disorder treatment programs offered me more of the same that had failed me each time. I now also believed, despite heated exchanges with my family, that I could never go back into hospital as I was now too fat to do so. I continued to survive despite innumerable odds and learned to keep myself from giving in completely to this debilitating illness that had taken so many lives to date. I had been through enough to have learned a great deal of information about functioning with the severity of illness that I have. From knowing my body cues and pushing myself to take medications to reduce the intensity of my symptoms of anxiety and compulsive rituals, I managed to survive and to continue with the albeit exceptionally poor quality of life that I endured on a daily basis.

My parents then discovered the harm reduction model, which has not only had a profound impact on my life but given me that glimpse of hope for the first time in almost three decades. I would be the first to assert that this form of treatment is not beneficial for most; I felt as though it has and can save my life. I needed a pathway, an opportunity to slowly but surely progress with weight gain whilst having to deal with an almost impenetrable fortress of ruminating thoughts conspiring to undermine every stride that I would take. The harm reduction model has afforded me the opportunity to give me reprieve and space from eating disorder thoughts and behaviors. I now have the lucidity and capacity to put vital and necessary space between my anorexia nervosa thoughts/urges and acting upon them. I have worked hard in incorporating the act of thought/action fusion in my daily life so that I can gain clarity and independence from the prison of the eating disorder. This benefits me greatly in being able to separate my thinking about my behaviors and then acting upon them. Working with a team that has accepted that I can live and survive at a lower-than-normal weight and that has helped manage bowel function expectations and significantly lower my use of laxatives, but without the expectation that I fully stop using them, has allowed me to actually make some positive changes. They were clear with me and my family that this approach still carries huge risk for me. My family has been able to be more accepting and thus more supportive.

I need to be very clear that the harm reduction model is not a silver bullet and/or panacea and is not perfect. Relapse is always possible, but [the model's] strength lies at its core in reducing harm wherever possible. The theory that underlies this model is to minimize behaviors and the potential injury that can happen with pernicious and noxious eating disorders. Yes, I have had lapses with this model, and as I have previously argued, it is not perfect. However, an outstanding feature has been my ability to have made marked improvements for the longest periods yet and thereby reduce some of the harm that would inevitably have followed. I have been able to sustain some progress rather than [let] expectations of full recovery [throw] me back to unabated engagement with eating disorder behaviors. I have some hope and a better quality of life.

References

Arkell J, Robinson PH: A pilot case series using qualitative and quantitative methods: biological, psychological and social outcome in severe and enduring eating disorder (anorexia nervosa). Int J Eat Disord 41:650–656, 2008

Bamford B, Barras C, Sly R, et al: Eating disorders symptoms and quality of life: where should clinicians place their focus in severe and enduring anorexia nervosa? Int J Eat Disord 48:133–138, 2015

Brickman B, Rabinowitz VC, Karuza J, et al: Models of helping and coping. Am Psychol 37:368–384, 1982

Broomfield C, Stedal K, Touys S, Rhodes P: Labeling and defining severe and enduring anorexia nervosa. Int J Eat Disord 50:611–623, 2017

Caplan G: Principles of Prevention Psychiatry. Oxford, UK, Basic Books, 1964

Dawson L, Rhodes P, Touys S: The recovery model and anorexia nervosa. Aust NZ J Psychiatry 48:1009–1016, 2014

Eddy K, Tabri N, Thomas, JJ, et al: Recovery from anorexia nervosa at 22-year follow-up. J Clin Psychiatry 78:184–189, 2017

Fairburn CG, Cooper Z: The Eating Disorder Examination, in Binge Eating: Nature, Assessment and Treatment, 12th Edition. Edited by Fairburn CG, Wilson GT. New York, Guilford, 1993, pp 317–331

Hay P, Touyz S: Classification challenges in the field of eating disorders: can severe and enduring anorexia nervosa be defined? J Eat Disord 6:41, 2018

Hay P, Phil D, Cho K: A qualitative exploration on influences on the process of recovery from personal written accounts of people with anorexia nervosa. Women Health 53(7):730–740, 2013

Hay P, Chinn D, Forbes D, et al: Royal Australian and New Zealand College of Psychiatrists clinical practice guidelines for the treatment of eating disorders. Aust NZ J Psychiatry 48:977–1008, 2014

Kaplan AS, Buchanan S: Is there a role for palliative care in the management of treatment resistant chronic anorexia nervosa? Presented at the International Conference on Eating Disorders, Austin, TX, May 2012

Kaplan AS, Strober M: Severe and enduring anorexia nervosa: can risk of persisting illness be identified, and prevented, in young patients? Int J Eat Disord 52:478–480, 2019

Khalsa SS, Portnoff LC, McCurdy-McKinnon D, Feusner JD: What happens after treatment? A systematic review of relapse, remission, and recovery in anorexia nervosa. J Eat Disord 5:20, 2017

Lopez A, Yager J, Feinstein RE: Medical futility and psychiatry: palliative care and hospice care as a last resort in the treatment of refractory anorexia nervosa. Int J Eat Disord 43:372–377, 2010

Marlatt GA, Witkiewitz K: Update on harm-reduction policy and intervention research. Annu Rev Clin Psychol 6:591–606, 2010

Robinson PH: Severe and enduring eating disorders: recognition and management. Adv Psychiatr Treat 20:392–401, 2014

Strober M: Managing the chronic, treatment-resistant patient with anorexia nervosa. Int J Eat Disord 36:245–255, 2004

Touyz S, La Grange D, Lacey H, et al: Treating severe and enduring anorexia nervosa: a randomized controlled trial. Psychol Med 43:2501–2511, 2013

Weissman MM, Bothwell S: Assessment of social adjustment by patient self-report. Arch Gen Psychiatry 33:1111–1115, 1976

Westmoreland P, Mehler PS: Caring for patients with severe and enduring eating disorders (SEED): certification, harm reduction, palliative care, and the question of futility. J Psychiatr Pract 22:313–320, 2016

Wodak A: Harm reduction is now the mainstream global drug policy. Addiction 104:343–345, 2009

Wonderlich SA, Mitchell JE, Crosby RD, et al: Minimizing and treating chronicity in the eating disorders: a clinical overview. Int J Eat Disord 45:467–475, 2012

10

Eating Disorders and Palliative Care

Patricia Westmoreland, M.D.
Libby Erickson, D.O.
Ovidio Bermudez, M.D., FAAP, FSAHM, FAED, Fiaedp, C.E.D.S.

IT is well established that individuals with chronic, severe mental illnesses (e.g., schizophrenia, bipolar disorder, major depressive disorder) die approximately 20 years earlier than the general population. This is in part due to the side effects of medication, socioeconomic factors, and patients' ability to engage in risk factor modification or reduction. Patients with eating disorders (EDs) face unique challenges with regard to morbidity and mortality because their mental illness is strongly intertwined with the physical symptoms of their disorder. A severe and persistent ED, such as anorexia nervosa (AN), carries with it the burden of multiple physical ills and has a mortality rate second only to opioid abuse (Chesney et al. 2014). The longer an ED persists, the more severe the illness becomes and the greater the number of medical and psychiatric comorbidities and risk of death (Arcelus et al. 2011; Haus et al. 2011).

Despite these factors, there is optimism regarding the possibility of recovery late in the course of an ED. Although only a small percentage of people with EDs recover within the first 10 years of illness, a recent study demonstrated that two-thirds of patients with AN had recovered at 22-year follow-up (Eddy et al. 2017). Recovery in patients with AN thus appears to continue over a prolonged period of time. The authors of this study wrote, "Our findings that recovery remains possible even after long-term illness argue for active treatment rather than palliative care for most patients" (Eddy et al. 2017). Williams et al. (1998) also questioned the role of palliative care in patients with EDs for whom recovery is possible, even in cases of long-standing severe AN.

Despite optimism resulting from the study by Eddy et al. (2017), complete recovery is not probable for some patients given the extent of their morbidity. The traditional method of treatment (hospitalization with a goal of complete weight restoration) is often not workable for people who have already endured multiple lengthy hospitalizations without benefit. Such patients may be among those with chronic severe mental illness who, as described by Trachsel et al. (2016), are at risk of "either therapeutic neglect or overly aggressive care." These patients may request a harm reduction model directed toward maintaining a minimal level of function. This includes restoring weight to a minimally acceptable level to reduce the risk of imminent death while conceding that the person is at high risk of requiring hospital care for conditions that may lead to deterioration and death. Harm reduction is discussed in more detail in Chapter 9.

If a person with an ED is unable to accede to the terms of a harm reduction model (e.g., unable to maintain the weight necessary), palliative care may be considered. *Palliation* means preventing or relieving suffering for people facing a severe or life-threatening illness. Palliative care as well as hospice care have been described as low-intensity treatments for patients with severe and enduring eating disorders (SEEDs) for whom a "cure" is unlikely as well as intolerable (Yager 2020).

Basic Tenets of Palliative Care

Palliative care is designed to improve the quality of life for patients with life-threatening illnesses, with the goal of reducing suffering through comfort care. Palliative care involves managing pain and symptoms, such as nausea and low energy levels, to optimize patients' quality of life as long as they remain alive. Although the term *palliative care* (i.e., symptomatic relief from pain or physical or mental stress) is not synonymous with *hospice care*, these terms are frequently conflated (Geppert 2015).

Palliative care does not necessarily mean "giving up" on life (Russon and Alison 1998) but means optimizing medical and psychiatric care for a person who has chosen palliation over cure. The World Health Organization (2020) defines *palliative care* as "the active care of patients whose disease is not responsive to curative treatment." This entails cooperation between palliative care specialists and other medical disciplines with the goal of decreasing the patient's physical and psychic pain (Trachsel et al. 2015). Patients with SEEDs who undergo palliative care are those for whom further treatment (be it with a goal of normalizing weight or achieving weight sufficient for harm reduction) is unlikely to resolve or decrease their illness and suffering.

Patients with SEEDs who elect palliative care often have untreatable comorbidities, either physical, such as renal or cardiac failure or severe osteoporosis, or psychological, such as severe treatment-refractory major depressive disorder or crippling anxiety. Symptomatic relief includes, but is not limited to, analgesics for pain associated with osteoporosis and stress fractures, wound care for decubitus ulcers, anxiolytics and antidepressant medications, and medications to improve sleep. The goal is for these individuals to be comfortable during the remainder of their life, albeit a shortened life. Continuing to treat them with the hope of returning them to an ideal body weight does more harm than good. Candidates for palliative care have usually had multiple prior treatments with no remission in their ED symptoms or any ability to sustain weight gain. By the time they begin considering palliative care, they are typically unable to accede to the terms necessary for a harm reduction model to work in their favor and a decision may have been made to forgo repeat hospitalizations and forced feeding (Trachsel et al. 2015).

The Academy for Eating Disorders (2016) has noted that, despite the potentially fatal consequences of an ED, full recovery is possible. However, it also recognizes the role of palliative care. There is also opposition to palliative and end-of-life care, with many professionals calling it a "slippery slope" that could result in all people with chronic EDs ending up in hospice or palliative care (Westmoreland and Mehler 2019).

Role of Psychiatry in Palliative Care of Severe and Enduring Eating Disorders

Aside from the treatment of anxiety and depression and its potential role in addressing grief and loss associated with palliative care, psychiatry is not traditionally included in palliative care. However, attention has shifted toward understanding chronic medical illnesses in patients with psychiatric problems and, with that, recognition of the role of psychiatry in palliative care. Interestingly, palliative care and psychiatry share significant overlap in clinical approach and origin in medicine. Both emerged from internal medicine and utilize a biopsychosocial model that frequently incorporates multidisciplinary teams (Trachsel et al. 2016). The collaboration between these fields has grown extensively and is typically referred to as "palliative care psychiatry" or "psycho-oncology." This collaborative specialty serves a diverse role addressing advance care planning, evaluating capacity, ruling out or treating delirium, and educating other medical professionals about appropriate palliative use of psychotropic medications (Bauer 2016). Advocating for patients and their families while at the same time trying to individualize treatment is also a vital component.

Addressing Advance Care Planning

When patients have a chronic psychiatric illness such as SEED, their clinical care is often paternalistic in nature, with little room for patient autonomy, even when they are capable of communicating a choice about their preferred care options. There is great disparity between the voice that people with mental illness wish they had and the voice they do have (i.e., proxy designation in the chart) (Foti 2003; Foti et al. 2005). Such disparity may be partially accounted for by social issues, such as lower rates of marriage in patients with severe psychiatric illness and estrangement from family, both of which are fairly prevalent in individuals with severe and enduring AN. They may also mistrust relatives involved in their care, especially when patient and family objectives are at odds (e.g., a patient with SEED eschewing weight restoration and family wanting a full course of treatment that includes weight restoration).

Perhaps partially because of concerns about differing goals and outcomes of treatment, the movement toward psychiatric advance directives has gained ground. In this manner, patients with SEEDs would be able to dictate their wishes regarding future treatment were they to decompensate. The advance directive, which is executed when patients are between acute episodes of care, theoretically spells out what they would or would not want in the event of acute illness. Topics addressed by a psychiatric advance directive include, but are not limited to, choice of hospital, choice of medications, and in the case of an ED, whether the person will accept tube feeding or compulsory treatment. Such were the tenants of a case in the United Kingdom. In *Local Authority v. E and Others* (2012), a patient with severe and chronic AN had previously executed two advance directives refusing compulsory feeding. Her parents and physicians argued that Ms. E was comparatively well when she executed the directives and requested that her wishes with regard to refusal of tube feeding be honored, even if it resulted in her death. The judge opined that Ms. E had cognitive distortions at the time of the hearing similar to those she had at the time she executed the directives. The judge ruled that the value of life trumps the presumption that further treatment will fail and ordered that she be involuntarily force fed. A critic of the judge's decision suggested that supporting the wishes of the patient and family may have been a better course of action than saving the life of someone who did not want to engage in further treatment and whose family supported her decision (Ryan and Callaghan 2014).

Individualizing Treatment

AN exists on a spectrum. There is a significant difference between, for example, a 14-year-old adolescent with an ED and a 40-year-old woman who has dealt with an ED for 25 years and been admitted to multiple treatment facilities (Touyz and Hay 2015). Measures of the quality of life with regard to the latter scenario are thought to be equal to the impairment of patients with schizophrenia or major depressive disorder (Robinson 2009). However, because the illness typically begins at a young age, it is not atypical for patients to die in their thirties, with a reported 5%–10% increase in death risk every decade thereafter (Steinhausen 2002).

Evaluating for Capacity

Psychiatric patients should execute an advance directive when their capacity is less in doubt. This decreases the likelihood that the directive will be challenged in court. However, determination of capacity can be challenging, especially in patients with EDs whose capacity (or lack thereof) is typically confined to the narrow area of food and body image. Chapter 4 deals in greater detail with evaluation of capacity.

There is debate as to whether clinical assessment versus an instrument-based assessment is best and whether capacity should be the ultimate determinant when deciding whether a person should engage in palliative care versus harm reduction or a full treatment course. A recent commentary asked that, even if such an individual did lack decisional capacity, then what? Should he or she be subjected to treatment that does more harm than good and has little or no hope of success? Surely this person has the capacity to assess the level of his or her own suffering, and perhaps that is more relevant to the question at hand (Yager 2015). There is also the question as to whether the quality of life among individuals with longstanding AN justifies the position of palliative care (Starzomska 2010). Draper (2000) noted that individuals with SEEDs such as AN can "neither live with the illness nor without it" and that people with a severe ED may choose palliative care not because they do not want to eat and get fat but rather because their quality of life is low and their suffering plentiful. Exhaustion, as a result of multiple years of illness, failed treatments, and medical complications, may also play a role in a person with AN requesting palliative care (Starzomska 2010).

A case in the United States dealt with a 30-year-old patient with a history of chronic AN in exactly this predicament. According to her treatment providers, forcing her into involuntary treatment or waiting for her to voluntarily engage in treatment was unlikely to cure her ED or even to afford her a reasonable quality of life (Lopez et al. 2010). Despite the termination of active care and initiation of hospice care, she was reluctant to discuss end-of-life issues and insisted that she would not and did not want to die, thus calling her competency into question. Her health continued to decline, and she died 3 weeks after admission to a hospice care unit. In another case review on the topic, patients who chose to succumb to their illness were elected to pursue end-of-life care (Campbell and Aulisio 2012). These patients were older than the patient described by Lopez et al. (2010), had longer periods of failed treatments, and their refusals of life-sustaining care had been consistent over a long period of time.

Ruling Out or Treating Delirium

By the time patients with SEEDs consider the possibility of palliative care, they are likely to have not only irremediable medical comorbidities but also cognitive features that, in an extreme state, may result in delirium. Delirium, entailing a fluctuating level of alertness, may be caused by medical complications of ED such as renal failure, heart failure, metabolic abnormalities, or certain medications (especially those that are anticholinergic in nature). Psychiatrists may be called upon in a palliative setting to diagnose delirium and provide treatment. A major part of treating delirium is identifying and rectifying the cause, whether that be removing an offending medication or treating a medical malady. Low-dose antipsychotics, such as haloperidol, risperidone, or quetiapine, may be useful adjuncts. Psychiatrists can educate treatment teams about administering psychiatric medication for the purposes of alleviating fear and anxiety as well as depression and, as previously noted, symptoms of delirium.

Psychiatrist as Advocate

The stigma of mental illness also extends to people with severe EDs when many professionals believe there is an automatic correlation between a mental illness such as a severe ED and incapacity. Such professionals may also feel uncomfortable caring for a person whose illness is thought to result from a volitional act (i.e., not eating, purging) rather than an illness such as cancer or heart failure. Respecting patient autonomy while relieving pain and suffering is an important principle common to both palliative care and psychiatry (Bauer 2016).

Dealing With Countertransference When Patients Request Palliative Care

Williams et al. (1998) noted, "when dealing with chronic illness, a doctor should be able to tolerate distress and negativism and still offer support as well as control of symptoms and effective treatment." They also noted that maintaining a positive therapeutic stance is paramount. However, this may be easier said than done with regard to an illness that claims most of its victims in the prime of their life. In addition to sharing expertise, sharing the burden of treating these patients between internal medicine and its ancillary disciplines as well as psychiatry may be helpful. The venue for palliative care should also be carefully considered (Russon and Alison 1998), and treatment either in the hospital or at home may be preferable depending on the circumstances.

Framework for Choosing Autonomy Over Paternalism

Some psychiatrists and ED professionals oppose palliative care, citing the "slippery slope" argument that would make all patients with SEED inherently eligible for end-of-life care. Proponents of this viewpoint argue that the illness compromises patients' ability to make a fully competent decision, and overriding their autonomy may be justified under the doctrine of paternalism in order to save their life and return them to a state at which they can make an informed and competent decision. ED professionals are justifiably reluctant to undertake any treatment that bears little hope of advancing a patient's quality of life, directly opposes the wishes of the patient and family, and simply extends a life of suffering, even if the patient has diminished capacity. Yet physicians are understandably also reluctant to give up hope. In addition, if a palliative care approach lessens the person's pain or anxiety/depression, that person may reach a point at which he or she is more likely to engage in the physical and psychotherapeutic work needed for recovery (Russon and Alison 1998). However, this hope should be balanced by careful assessment of each person's circumstances so that patients are not forced into an intolerable living situation merely because they are deemed to lack capacity. In addition, even if patients do not have decision-making capacity, they are likely still capable of appraising their own suffering (Kendall 2014; Yager 2015). A decision in favor of palliative care should be made on a case-by-case basis and applied when considering a particular treatment intervention, at a particular time, for a particular patient.

Several frameworks have been proposed that balance patients' wishes with concerns about those with impaired decision-making capacity refusing further treatment. Draper (2000) proposed respecting patients' autonomy if they have been affected "beyond the natural cycle of the disorder"—defined (in this instance) as 1–8 years. Other considerations she proposed in deciding not to override autonomy include not forcibly treating patients who have been force fed on previous occasions, respecting the wishes of patients who have insight into the effect AN has had on their lives, and preferring that patients not make decisions about care when they are close to death. Draper also argued that the decision made by individuals with severe and chronic AN to end their lives should be considered "on a par" with decisions to refuse life-prolonging care made by those with other chronic debilitating disorders. A proposed framework by McKinney (2015) denoted that decisions about further episodes of care should be made at a time when patients are competent (i.e., ideally between episodes). These individuals must know that refusing nutrition will lead to their death, and their decision to embark on a course of palliative care must be based on a realistic assessment of their current quality of life and the low probability that current or future treatment will succeed. They must also be consistent in communicating their desires.

Case Example

C.B. was a 43-year-old female with a history of AN, binge-purging type. She had first presented for treatment at age 15, when her restrictive patterns began. Subsequently, she has had numerous rounds of treatment at varying levels of care, including inpatient, residential, and partial hospitalization, and has required certification for involuntary treatment on several occasions. C.B. currently presents at a weight of 79 lb (height 5 ft 6 in; 60% of ideal body weight) and has various stress fractures due to excessive exercise and osteoporosis, metabolic abnormalities, and renal insufficiency. She experiences high amounts of pain and has incapacitating anxiety with dissociative episodes and a depressed mood. C.B. was placed on a hold for grave disability, and a nasogastric tube was initiated.

Co-occurring PTSD and major depressive disorder have complicated C.B.'s treatment. Both conditions have been minimally responsive to an assortment of treatments, including many psychotropic medication trials, electroconvulsive therapy, and most recently intranasal ketamine. Throughout the progression of her illness, she has maintained a high level of achievement, including completing a college degree at a large university out of state as well as a law degree at a prestigious university. Despite these intellectual feats and her capacity in other domains, C.B. has maintained cognitive distortions regarding body image and food throughout her adult life.

During several treatments, C.B. was able to fully restore weight but, with time, would relapse, lose the weight, and return to treatment either voluntarily or involuntarily. On several occasions between treatment stays she expressed a desire to avoid future involuntary treatments and nasogastric feeds and to remain at home for treatment to allow her to continue her personal endeavors. C.B. voiced these desires at times when she was weight-restored and appeared cognitively intact.

At her most recent admission, C.B. and her family voiced her desire to engage in voluntary treatment to restore her weight and interrupt her binge and purge behaviors. Appreciating C.B.'s articulated preference about treatment, nasogastric tube feeding and the mental health hold were terminated. The team decided not to pursue another court order for involuntary treatment. C.B. restored her weight to 101 lb and achieved some relief of her trauma symptoms and depression with continued intranasal ketamine treatments and individual and family psychotherapy. Her goal, along with her medical team, became one of harm reduction, and they agreed she would maintain her weight at 100 lb in an effort to see if that would be more tolerable and sustainable for her.

Following discharge, C.B. returned to work as an attorney despite not being fully weight-restored. She was active with her friend group and spent time with family. However, she was unable to maintain her weight and required three more hospitalizations to regain the weight lost and return to the 100-lb goal. Despite the harm reduction plan in place, she continued to engage in excessive amounts of exercise and other compensatory behaviors, running upward of 2 hours daily and relying on vomiting and laxatives as compensatory purging behaviors when she did eat. Her weight dropped to 78 lb, and she was encouraged to return to treatment, given fear of her history of severe medical complications.

C.B. determined with her outpatient team that returning to treatment would be futile, given its ineffectiveness in restoring her weight and her inability to engage in a harm reduction approach to care. After 28 years of treatment, C.B.'s AN was deemed treatment resistant. C.B. received weekly therapy that was not specific to her ED, and appointments were void of weigh-ins and discussions of caloric intake. She continued psychiatric follow-up and received medication for both her mood and trauma symptoms as well as pain management for her several physical ailments. The team agreed on no ED interventions unless requested by the patient.

C.B.'s weight continued to trend downward, her restrictive behaviors and exercise continued, and she ultimately was unable to work and only minimally able to leave home. No further interventions were provided beyond what she requested. C.B. passed away 3 weeks later from cardiac complications secondary to her AN.

Conclusion

Every case must be considered in a nuanced and thoughtful manner. For patients with SEEDs, clinicians must realistically assess the patients' capacity for recovery or ability to engage in a harm reduction or palliative care model. At the same time, clinicians must remain in touch with the wishes of patients, their families, and the treatment team and consider the burden on caregivers and stewardship over expenditure of health care resources when deciding whether to recommend traditional (whether voluntary or involuntary), harm reduction, palliative, or end-of-life care. Clinicians should arrive at that decision only after an extensive and well-considered decision-making process. Failing to consider end-of-life care as an option for patients with a chronic and severe psychiatric illness such as AN may perpetuate the stigma of mental illness as separate from physical illness and force a small but noteworthy group of patients into an intolerable situation.

References

Academy for Eating Disorders: The Academy for Eating Disorders advocates for early intervention and specialized care for eating disorders in response to Morristown, NJ ruling. Newswise, December 15, 2016

Arcelus J, Mitchell AJ, Wales J, Nielsen S: Mortality rates in patients with anorexia nervosa and other eating disorders: a meta-analysis of 36 studies. Arch Gen Psychiatry 68:724–731, 2011

Bauer RL: Ethical considerations regarding end-of-life planning and palliative care needs in patients with chronic psychiatric disorders. Am J Psychiatry Resid J 11(5):4–6, 2016

Campbell AT, Aulisio MP: The stigma of "mental illness": end stage anorexia and treatment refusal. Int J Eat Disord 45:627–634, 2012

Chesney E, Goodwin GM, Fazel S: Risks of all-cause and suicide mortality in mental disorders: a meta-review. World Psychiatry 13(2):153–160, 2014

Draper H: Anorexia nervosa and respecting a refusal of life-prolonging therapy: a limited justification. Bioethics 14(2):120–133, 2000

Eddy KT, Tabri N, Thomas JJ, et al: Recovery from anorexia nervosa and bulimia nervosa at 22-year follow-up. J Clin Psychiatry 78(2):184–189, 2017

Foti ME: "Do it your way": a demonstration project on end-of-life care for patients with serious mental illness. J Pall Med 6:661–669, 2003

Foti ME, Bartels SJ, Merriman MP, et al: Medical advance directive planning for persons with serious mental illness. Psychiatr Serv 56:576–584, 2005

Geppert CMA: Futility in chronic anorexia nervosa: a concept whose time has not yet come. Am J Bioethics 15(7):34–43, 2015

Haus C, Caille A, Godart N, et al: Factors predictive of ten-year mortality in severe anorexia nervosa patients. Acta Psychiatr Scand 123:62–70, 2011

Kendall S: Anorexia nervosa: the diagnosis. J Bioeth Inq 11:31–40, 2014

Local Authority v. E and others, EWHC 1639 (COP), 2012 COPLR 441

Lopez A, Yager J, Feinstein RE: Medical futility and psychiatry: palliative care and hospice care as a last resort in the treatment of refractory anorexia nervosa. Int J Eat Disord 43:372–377, 2010

McKinney C: Is resistance (n)ever futile? A response to "Futility in chronic anorexia nervosa: a concept whose time has not yet come" by Cynthia Geppert. Am J Bioethics 15:47–50, 2015

Robinson P: Severe and Enduring Eating Disorder (SEED): Management of Complex Presentations of Anorexia and Bulimia Nervosa. Chichester, UK, John Wiley and Sons, 2009

Russon L, Alison D: Does palliative care have a role in treatment of anorexia nervosa? Palliative care does not mean giving up. BMJ 317(7152):196–197, 1998

Ryan CJ, Callaghan S: Treatment refusal in anorexia nervosa: the hardest cases. J Bioeth Inq 11:43–45, 2014

Starzomska M: Controversial issues concerning the concept of palliative care of anorexic patients. Arch Psychiatry Psychother 4:49–50, 2010

Steinhausen HC: The outcome of anorexia nervosa in the 20th century. Am J Psychiatry 159:1294–1303, 2002

Touyz S, Hay P: Severe and enduring anorexia nervosa (SE-AN): in search of a new paradigm. J Eat Disord 3:26, 2015

Trachsel M, Wild V, Biller-Andorno N, Krones T: Compulsory treatment in chronic anorexia nervosa by all means? Searching for a middle ground between a curative and palliative approach. Am J Bioeth 15(7):55–56, 2015

Trachsel M, Irwin SI, Biller-Andorno N, et al: Palliative care psychiatry for severe and persistent mental illness. Lancet 3:100, 2016

Westmoreland P, Mehler P: Eating disorders and palliative care, in Gürze/Salucore Eating Disorders Resource Catalogue (website), January 27, 2019. Available at: https://www.edcatalogue.com/eating-disorders-palliative-care. Accessed February 2019.

Williams J, Pieri L, Sims A: Does palliative care have a role in the treatment of anorexia nervosa? BMJ 317:195–197, 1998

World Health Organization: WHO definition of palliative care. WHO website, 2020. Available at: https://www.who.int/cancer/palliative/definition/en. Accessed August 8, 2020.

Yager J: The futility of arguing about medical futility in anorexia nervosa: the question is how you would handle highly specific circumstances. Am J Bioeth 15(7):47–50, 2015

Yager J: Managing patients with severe and enduring eating disorders: when is enough, enough? J Nerv Ment Dis 208(4):277–282, 2020

11

Futility

Cynthia M.A. Geppert, M.D., M.A., M.P.H., M.B.E., D.P.S., M.S.J, FACLP, DFAPA, FASAM, HEC-C
Joel Yager, M.D.
Jeanne Kerwin, D.M.H., HEC-C

Futility: History and Definitions

Medicine has recognized the concept of "futility" since the time of Hippocrates. Hippocrates wrote from the perspective of a paternalistic model of medicine in which physicians, despite or because of their limited scientific knowledge, wielded the power to determine when treatment was futile and should be unilaterally withheld (Reiser et al. 1977). In the 1960s, research abuses and aggressive use of newly developed life-sustaining technologies contributed to a new model of patient self-determination. In this "autonomy" model of medicine, patients and their surrogates evaluate the options available to them and may at times request modalities of treatment that medical professionals believe to be "futile."

The modern definition of *futility* has been the subject of clinical and philosophical debate. In an effort to clarify its meaning, Schneiderman et al. (1990), Pope (2012), and others have described different types. *Physiological futility* occurs when an intervention simply cannot achieve its clinical goals (e.g., cardiopulmonary resuscitation in a patient with a ruptured ventricle) and is the domain in which medical decision making is based on the technical knowledge available at the time. *Quantitative futility* relies on empirical evidence that a treatment has not benefited patients in the past 100 similar cases. Ethicists who support nonphysiological futility contend that physicians need not offer treatments that only maintain a patient in an unresponsive state or continued reliance on intensive care.

Qualitative futility assesses the burdens and benefits of a proposed treatment relative to achieving a values-driven goal. When practitioners determine that the risks or burdens outweigh the benefits, they may not have an ethical obligation to offer them. Some ethicists have criticized these latter two types as value judgments masked as clinical determinations, emphasizing that only patients or their surrogates can weigh benefits and burdens in accordance with their own personal values and goals of care. Contemporary ethicists and practitioners advocate jettisoning the "futility" terminology in favor of less values-laden and more accessible terms such as "potentially inappropriate" or "nonbeneficial." These new formulations, as detailed in the 2015 American Thoracic Society policy (Bosslet et al. 2015), underscore that aggressive use of lifesaving technology at the end of a patient's life may not only fail to realize that patient's goals of care but also cause actual harm.

The classic futility dilemma involves a patient or surrogate insisting on treatment that practitioners believe to be nonbeneficial, but there are also situations in which clinicians or, in some eating disorder (ED) cases, the courts demand treatment that medical professionals consider inappropriate. These "reverse futility" dilemmas are one example of the complexities that emerge when futility is transposed from the field of medicine to psychiatry and in particular to EDs. This new application of the concept requires an intensive examination of ethical issues that arise in an area in which uncertain prognosis, competing best interests, and the presumed primacy of a patient's preferences and values make evaluation of benefits, burdens, and harms particularly perplexing.

Does "End-Stage" Anorexia Exist?

Historically, futility disputes revolved around patients in the latter phase of their disease process, such as the patient with metastatic cancer or heart failure to whom physicians refer as "end-stage." We are only beginning to explore whether psychiatric disorders have a corresponding "end-stage" and, if so, how it would be characterized. This lack of knowledge confounds discussions of futility for individuals with psychiatric illness and their families and surrogates.

End-stage disease, or terminal illness, usually refers to the last, irreversible phase in the course of a progressive disease, when no evidence-based medical interventions are known or available to aid recovery and life is unlikely to be sustained for long (e.g., no more than 3–6 months) without extraordinary external medical interventions (e.g., chronic dialysis or other forms of life support) (Buzgova et al. 2017; Tripodoro and De Vito 2015). At this stage, clinicians usually focus on providing comfort care. Although the term "end-stage" has appeared in the anorexia nervosa (AN) literature (Campbell and Aulisio 2012; Gans and Gunn 2003), there is no consensus as to the definition of end-stage AN, and no studies have yet estimated the percentage of patients with AN who progress to end-stage status. On the basis of our clinical experience, we endorse the observation that such states do exist but that they probably occur no more frequently than in 5% of patients with AN. (For example, in a career involving the care of hundreds of patients with EDs, J.Y. has seen only 5–10 such patients.)

Although the research into end-stage AN is just beginning, there is increasing evidence that some cases are better classified as severe and enduring eating disorders (SEEDs) (Robinson 2009). This definition emerged in the literature to describe a condition that is present when a patient has had signs, symptoms, and impairments related to AN that have persisted for many years (Robinson et al. 2015; Touyz and Hay 2015). Although these conditions are also sometimes referred to as "severe and enduring anorexia nervosa," SEED-AN, or SEAN, we use SEED in this chapter.

Around 20% of patients with AN are considered to have a SEED. Although no absolute duration has been determined for this designation, some ED treatment experts consider the condition to be present when a patient has sustained illness for as little as 6 years, whereas others use the term only after a patient has been ill for at least 10–12 years. Although recovery is not impossible at this point, and patients with AN may recover after many years of illness, the odds of complete recovery appear to be slim. Individuals with SEEDs have a chronic illness of long duration that is, for the most part, progressive and unremitting. Concerns about labeling patients with SEED are well intentioned, because clinicians and families fear generating self-fulfilling prophecies regarding poor outcomes—that is, they fear patients who are labeled as having a chronic illness will more readily adopt the role of chronicity, give up hope, and exert less effort to get better. However, failure to realistically acknowledge that person's status can also lead to unrealistic expectations or pressures for recovery, leading to experiences of defeat for patients, families, and clinicians, with accompanying guilt, shame, anguish, feelings of failure, and considerable waste of resources. Patients with SEEDs may sustain themselves nutritionally for years, especially if their ED involves restrictive behavior rather than bingeing and purging, the consequences of which may be less predictable. Even though they are undernourished, they eat just enough to keep getting by. At the same time, they may slowly and progressively accumulate medical complications related to undernutrition (e.g., cognitive slowing, gastroparesis, osteoporosis).

For some patients with SEEDs, such as the young women in the cases detailed at the end of this chapter, additional complications may come in the form of comorbid psychiatric or medical conditions, including mood, anxiety, personality, and substance use disorders; the effects of subclinical or clinical states of malnutrition; and other intercurrent medical conditions. At some point, for some patients, these vulnerabilities may push them over the tipping point to what would be considered end-stage disease.

What Characterizes Patients With End-Stage Anorexia Nervosa?

In our experience, the key features that distinguish individuals with severe, chronic, reasonably stable AN from those who have reached their tipping point are usually psychological. Because the willingness and ability to take in the minimum amount of nutrition necessary to sustain life and function is a *sine qua non* for survival, the absence of willingness or ability to take in nutrients by mouth or tube feeding, accompanied by rejection of the recommendations of treatment professionals, augurs end-stage conditions.

What distinguishes patients with prolonged illness from those in early onset and acute stages of AN who are unwilling or unable to make necessary efforts to imbibe nutrition? In earlier onset acute cases of shorter duration, assertive imposed interventions may be lifesaving and precede good improvement (Schreyer et al. 2016; Westmoreland et al. 2017). However, when patients are older, have been struggling ineffectively for decades, and appear to have decisional capacity, long-term refusal of nutrition becomes more complex. Patients may lose their will to live or to fight their disease for a variety of reasons, some judicious and others capricious, some malleable and others fixed. Here, little evidence has shown that ongoing treatment will alter their illness course (Yager 2007). The bottom line is that, unless the motivation and minimum ability to nourish oneself remains, patients with SEED who "throw in the towel" can be thought of as entering end-stage disease.

It is at this juncture that clinical decisions must include ethical analysis and recommendations, especially regarding three key issues: futility, capacity, and palliative care. Three crucial questions face these patients and their family/surrogates. We have based these questions, discussed in the sections that follow, on our own experience as clinicians and ethicists, as well as on the literature we consider relevant in answering them.

Does Futility Apply to Severe and Enduring Eating Disorders?

The concept of "futility" in medical care ordinarily addresses the futility of further treatment, signifying that no other evidence-based treatments are available to offer. It has been argued that no such treatments exist that reverse chronic or, certainly, end-stage AN (Yager 2015). Alternately, it has been noted that almost all medical complications of a severe ED are reversible with adequate nutrition (Westmoreland et al. 2017). Although we lack evidence about whether and how often restoring full nutritional health, voluntarily or involuntarily, will alter the cognition of patients with SEEDs to the point that they might be ready to give up the disorder, clinical experience suggests such transformations are rarely likely to occur, if ever. However, even if rare, if this reversibility extends to the cognitive distortions and lack of insight that perpetuate the ED so that patients regain a capacity to voluntarily engage in treatment, then it becomes more difficult to apply the classic medical concept of futility, and the ethical warrant for continuing treatment is thus stronger.

If one takes the position that nutritional treatment is not futile and can at least maintain life in chronically ill food-refusing, help-rejecting patients (up to and including involuntary feeding), clinicians face a different set of ethical issues. Here, even when families and clinicians desire to intervene against patients' wishes, challenges arise via numerous conflicting ethical perspectives (autonomy vs. beneficence and nonmaleficence) and medicolegal barriers (imposing long-term involuntary status on patients who may reasonably be said to have decisional capacity). There are also practical roadblocks, for example, locating and paying for institutions and staff that are willing to treat and capable of treating long-term involuntary patients who require tube feedings, and the fact that no current intervention has shown long-term evidence-based effectiveness. Another roadblock to care entails avoiding financial conflicts and other perverse incentives involving staff and families, such as the imposition or "selling" by provider organizations of costly treatments with unproven long-term benefit, and the acting out of conscious or unconscious anger by frustrated families and staff toward vulnerable patients through harsh, punitive behavioral programs of questionable value. When no professionals or institutions are available, willing, or able to treat such patients and no funds are available to sustain such treatments, what does one do? In such cases, decision-making that argues for maintaining life at any cost comes up short compared with more realistic (and possibly ethical) paths offered by "consequence-based decision-making" (Yager 2015).

As the chapter introduction demonstrates, futility is a concept in search of a definition, or as Ron Pies (2015) opined, both futility and the construct of end-stage psychiatric disorders are "category errors." A *category error* is a type of logical fallacy in which the qualities of one entity are attributed to another to which they do not apply. In this case, the medical concepts of end-stage disorders and futility are mistakenly applied to a psychiatric disorder—AN. Clinical judgments about patients with SEED being end-stage do not have the same physiologically based diagnostic and prognostic signs and symptoms as other recognized end-stage conditions such as heart failure and chronic obstructive pulmonary disease.

We have reviewed some studies showing that patients with SEEDs have a low likelihood of responding to any available treatments, yet found no conclusive evidence this is true. In addition, no reliable diagnostic prognostic signs and symptoms of end-stage AN have been identified to which the concept of futility might apply. In cases of multiorgan failure and metastatic cancers, we can accurately say that no effective treatment in the scientific armamentarium will forestall progression of these maladies, much less reverse their course. This is not true of SEEDs until the final few days of the patient's life, by which time medical professionals are dealing with terminal physiological processes, not with an ED. Prior to these final few days, however, the possibility, albeit remote, exists that this patient may respond to treatment after decades of illness and multiple therapeutic failures. In contrast, no one with metastatic cancer ever recovers, short of a miracle.

With regard to the cost of treating SEEDs, the long-term treatment is emotionally exhausting for families, defeating for health care professionals, and a huge and low-yield investment of scarce resources. However, the same can be said of many other medical and psychiatric disorders, such as chronic pain and addiction. It is ethically problematic to make treatment decisions on the basis of these barriers and burdens, even in a country that fails to provide health care for its most disabled citizens or fails in its quest to establish a system of just health care allocation.

Do Patients With SEEDs Have Decisional Capacity to Forgo Life-Sustaining Treatment?

The short answer to this complex question (as detailed in Chapter 5) is that some do and some do not have capacity. Some patients have been around the block many times and know that they are unable to continue fighting their eating-disordered thoughts, that despite many well-intentioned treatments they are unlikely to improve, and that they have little to no quality of life and none to look forward to. They are also aware of their extreme psychic pain and the consequences of not agreeing to treatments that support and prolong life. Many of these patients simply disengage from treatment, do not show up for appointments, and sign out of inpatient or residential treatment against medical advice. In this way, they resemble patients with chronic renal disease who elect not to continue hemodialysis, or those with chronic alcohol use disorder who opt to avoid treatment and drink themselves to death. Few clinicians would seek or wish to impose long-term involuntary treatment on these patients. Imposing involuntary treatment on a person with SEED simply to sustain life's physiological processes may not be ethically justifiable unless the clinician can honestly expect the outcome to offer a reasonable chance of meaningful recovery with acceptable quality of life. For example, consider how clinicians approach patients with end-stage dementia.

An argument may be made that when a patient's incapacity is due to extreme malnutrition, a time-limited trial of even involuntary treatment with the express goal of restoring decision-making capacity can be ethically justified. Patients with delirium tremens would not likely be considered capable of refusing acute treatment for life-threatening withdrawal. Once their delirium resolved, however, they could refuse further treatment for alcohol use disorder, just as patients with SEEDs who regain capacity can decline ongoing therapy for their ED. Of course, some patients with SEEDs refuse treatment based on the delusional idea that even small amounts of nutrition necessary to sustain life will make them fat. If the chances are reasonable that these delusions and the course of illness might be reversed by active interventions, clinicians and families might make a case for some period of involuntary treatment. However, if clinicians are unable to reasonably expect interventions will reverse psychiatric causes contributing to impaired decision making, imposing involuntary treatment on patients with SEEDs is ethically questionable.

Critics point out that this line of reasoning, though it has a compelling pragmatic rationale, begs the question of mental capacity. Conceding that some patients with SEED may have decisional capacity regarding treatment whereas others clearly do not, this is an important component of dealing with this population. Lack of mental capacity in patients with EDs can be attributed to malnutrition, delusions, a thought disorder, or executive dysfunction. The reality is that we are only beginning to understand what goes wrong in the cognitive, affective, and volitional processes of AN. This suggests two reasons to be cautious about endorsing futility, even in SEEDs. The first is that new research may find that patients whom conventional cognitive criteria identify as having decision-making capacity actually have emotional impairment that functionally renders them incapable. Second, research may lead to new, more promising treatment approaches that improve the chances these people can make meaningful therapeutic progress (Steinglass and Foerde 2018).

Is Palliative Care Appropriate in Futile Cases?

In our view, when other treatments are futile, palliative care is an excellent compassionate alternative (Lopez et al. 2010). Indeed, good palliative care incorporates all the elements of supportive care likely to benefit many individuals by reducing the conflicting goals and expectations of patients and staff, reducing the sense that either patients or staff are "failing" at their roles, and providing patients with easier, more relaxed alliances with their caregivers. J.Y. has seen several patients with SEEDs enter palliative care and thereafter demonstrate a greater degree of clinical stability in the ensuing months than had been the case in the months leading up to palliative care. By removing pressures and conflicts inherent to traditional ED treatment, individuals with SEEDs may be able to better relax into stable chronicity (see Chapters 9 and 10). Alternatively, patients who ultimately die through this process are at least able to do so on their own terms, without being subject to treatments that might have prolonged their lives but been neither curative, comforting, nor in their best interests.

In the Matter of A.G.

On February 20, 2017, a young woman known as A.G. died in the palliative care unit of a New Jersey hospital 3 months after a court decision that allowed her to forgo further forced treatments for her SEED. A.G. had been offered a range of treatments in various settings over the preceding 20 years. She had either eloped from or refused treatment and had experienced no sustained periods of remission. In 2014, she was involuntarily committed to a state psychiatric hospital after being found unconscious from using alcohol and sedatives in what was assumed to have been a suicide attempt. During her 2-year stay in that facility, she completed a Physician's Orders for Life-Sustaining Treatment (POLST) form with her clinician and stated her goals as "I want to live freely and not being bothered by anyone." The POLST included do not intubate, do not resuscitate, and do not administer artificial nutrition orders as well as a request for no further hospitalizations.

A.G.'s condition continued to worsen until her weight loss, multiple fractures, and new-onset seizures compelled the facility to obtain a temporary guardian and transfer A.G. to an acute-care hospital in June 2016. The court orders were "to obtain and/or procure any and all medical treatment for A.G., including, but not limited to, life-saving treatment and/or force feeding by any medical means, and/or intubation and the insertion of a

PEG tube" (*In the matter of A.G.* 2016). A.G. was then admitted to the intensive care unit weighing 65 lb and prescribed total parenteral nutrition. Despite psychiatric interventions, she continued to binge and purge and remained agitated, angry, and violent about being force fed. After suffering severe congestive heart failure requiring further interventions, total parenteral nutrition was discontinued, and A.G. refused any further forced treatments. Her weight plummeted back to the 60- to 70-lb range.

The New Jersey Department of Human Services, Division of Mental Health and Addiction Services submitted a motion opposing the request of A.G.'s guardian to change the orders to palliative care. On November 2, 2016, the Superior Court of New Jersey began hearings on the case. Testimony was heard from all interested parties, including A.G., who, due to her fragile physical state, testified before the judge and attorneys in her hospital unit. On November 21, 2016, Judge Paul W. Armstrong's ruling reiterated the legal rights and ethical principles articulated in landmark cases such as *Quinlan* and *Cruzan* and the hospital ethics opinion submitted in this case as founding support for A.G.'s request. He wrote,

> Here the esteemed legal canon of our State Supreme Court and the United States Supreme Court informs and authenticates the compassionate process followed by A.G.'s family and caregivers and impels this court to grant the uniform prayer of her legal guardian and legal counsel to authorize the provision of palliative care to A.G. as incident to her best interest. (*In the matter of A.G.* 2016).

A.G. requested palliative care, supported by her parents, guardian, and medical teams. A bioethics consultation was requested to analyze the following unique questions:

- Could a patient with an ED have the capacity to decide to forgo artificial feeding and transition to a palliative care plan?
- Was there a defined "end-stage" to an ED?
- What were the treatment options, and would they cause more suffering and harm to the patient than sustainable benefit?
- Could the application of forced feeding against the patient's vigorous refusals be deemed to be futile treatment?

After extensive discussion with the treating psychiatrists and medical team and a review of recent relevant literature (Lopez et al. 2010), the ethical consultant made the following recommendations:

1. There is clear recognition in law and ethics that competent adults have the right to refuse medical treatment, including life-sustaining treat-

ment, and those with a psychiatric disorder must not automatically be excluded from this basic right (Campbell and Aulisio 2012). Although the courts had involuntarily committed A.G. to a psychiatric facility, her psychiatric and medical teams subsequently assessed her as having decision-making capacity regarding treatment options.

2. There was no consensus in the literature that clearly answered the question as to whether A.G.'s ED could be defined as end-stage. However, based on the literature reviewed, A.G.'s lengthy ED history did not predict the possibility of sustained recovery, and many features of her ED indicated poor prognosis.

3. Forced life-saving treatments were antithetical to A.G.'s clearly stated goals but could potentially extend her life. The clinical team reviewed all treatment options, but after considering the physical, psychological, and emotional harms to her, they deemed them inhumane, not sustainable, and ethically unacceptable. Palliative care could provide A.G. with management of her physical discomfort as well as ongoing psychiatric care and emotional support. It was the only intervention that stood any reasonable chance of ameliorating her suffering and providing benefit, whether that benefit would be a desire for recovery or support on a path toward a peaceful and comfortable death.

4. *Futility* is strictly defined as those treatments that cannot achieve the desired clinical effect. Thus, life-sustaining treatments for A.G. could not be categorically defined as futile. The focus of ethical concern in this case was *not* futility but rather the significant harm to A.G. from forced treatments, the nonsustainable benefit to her, and the ultimate respect for her values and self-determination.

The ethics opinion thus recorded in her medical record held that the most compassionate, humane, and medically appropriate care plan was allowing A.G. to transition to palliative care with continued psychiatric treatments, medical management of pain and other physical symptoms, and maximum psychological, emotional, and spiritual support for her and her family.

In the Matter of S.A.

S.A. had had severe AN since age 13 and reached a crisis point in June 2017, when she was 20 years old, after she collapsed in her family home. She was admitted to an acute care hospital weighing just 60 lb and was stabilized and transferred to an ED center in Princeton, New Jersey, where she underwent treatment, including artificial tube feeding. Her psychiatrist and medical doctors were of the opinion that she was delusional, in denial, and did not understand her risk of dying and thus did not have the capacity to make her own medical decisions. S.A.'s parents wished to override their daughter's refusal of treatment and provide compulsory feedings in an effort to save her life. S.A. articulated her wishes to return home and manage her own ED and described being in treatment as "torture." She said she would choose death over treatment, according to the judge.

Judge Armstrong, who had also rendered the opinion in the case of A.G. (*In the matter of A.G.* 2016), again showing deference to taking S.A.'s testimony in person in her inpatient setting, concluded that her parents were acting in her best interest to save her life and that she had neither reached the same stage of organ failure and grave functional debility as A.G. nor had endured as many years of failed inpatient treatment (*In the matter of S.A.* 2017). In his decision, he granted the parents guardianship over her medical decisions in the hope that S.A. could have some beneficial outcome from further treatment.

This case is arguably different from that of A.G., in which the judge's decision allowed her to choose a palliative care approach. A.G. had failed to gain any sustainable benefit from treatments over the previous 15 years, remained opposed to treatment, and had severe physical debility, bone fractures, skin wounds, and organ failures (*In the matter of A.G.* 2016); S.A. had not reached a stage of multiorgan failure in which recovery would be highly improbable and did not have the same chronic serious disabilities (*In the matter of S.A.* 2017). A.G.'s treating psychiatrist, medical doctor, bioethics consultants, medical guardian, and parents had all supported her right to forgo further treatments against her wishes and had not believed she had any realistic chance of recovery, leaving palliative care the most humane choice. However, those interested parties in the case of S.A., most importantly her parents, did not agree with her decision and believed she had a higher likelihood of responding to aggressive treatment.

Local Authority vs. E and Others

Like A.G., E was an engaging, gifted woman. Ironically, she had once studied to be a doctor. Alcohol and opioid use disorder, as well as borderline personality disorder secondary to childhood sexual abuse, complicated her clinical course. On May 18, 2012, the local authority where she lived in the United Kingdom applied to the court of protection, requesting her case be urgently examined due to her extremely compromised state. E had been refusing to eat for the past 2 months and was drinking only small amounts of water. At the time the court was asked to intervene, E, at the age of 32 and with a BMI of 11.3, had been in a community hospital receiving hospice care for 5 weeks.

Like many patients with EDs, E had tried and failed many treatments over decades of care, including being detained under Britain's Mental Health Act on as many as 10 occasions. She reported not wanting to die but seeing no point in living, having spent most of her twenties in institutions. A somewhat unique facet of this case was that E had twice attempted to complete advance decision documents that would enable her to refuse life-sustaining treatment. Her parents and primary physicians opposed another trial of forced feeding because it would rob her of any control or dignity. The local authorities took a neutral stance but agreed to abide by the court's ruling (*Local Authority vs. E and Others* 2012).

At the court hearing in May 2012, the judge cited as persuasive several of the clinical ethics considerations raised in the counterpoint sections of this chapter. He opined that although E was very sick, she was not incurable, and that the preservation of life in a young, sapient person was ethically a *prima facie* principle and reflected a long legal tradition of protecting the sanctity of life (*Local Authority vs. E and Others* 2012). The judge concluded that Ms. E lacked capacity to refuse life-sustaining treatment for her ED precisely *because* of her ED. "However, there is strong evidence that E's obsessive fear of weight gain makes her incapable of weighing the advantages and disadvantages of eating in any meaningful way" (*Local Authority vs. E and Others* 2012).

Judge Jackson underscored that even experts could not agree about E's capacity, and no formal assessment of her mental capacity had been documented at the time the forms were completed. He considered this dearth of consensus and clear evaluation regarding such an irreversible decision to be dispositive and ruled that E did not have capacity when she completed the form refusing life-sustaining treatment including feeding. These conclusions left the court only two equally difficult interpretations of the best interest standard: permit E to die or constrain her to be fed. The decision forthrightly recognized the risks of refeeding and the low prospect of benefit (estimated at 20%) as well as the traumatizing effect of restraint and force. However, the judge identified two more compelling arguments: that no expert could say recovery was impossible with treatment and that, even if treatment could not restore Ms. E to a bearable quality of life, it might sufficiently improve her condition to allow her to regain the capacity to make her own decision (*Local Authority vs. E and Others* 2012).

To our knowledge, and contrary to the case of A.G., an expert ethics opinion was neither sought nor rendered in this case. Three primary ethical-legal questions were put to Judge Jackson, all of which centered around decision-making capacity. The first was whether Ms. E, at the time of the hearing, had the mental capacity to autonomously refuse the forced feeding necessary to save her life. The second was whether she had possessed mental capacity when she executed her advance decision documents refusing life-sustaining treatments, even if she lacked mental capacity now, and if such a refusal was applicable under the current circumstances. If she *had* been capable, then a decision regarding her treatment refusal could have been made on the basis of substituted judgment. Finally, if E was incapable in both instances, then what was in her best interests?

Ms. E, her solicitors, physicians, advocates, and parents held that even if she had lost her mental capacity to make decisions about her ED, she had not lost the right to make a decision to die when she believed further treatment would not be beneficial. She had, they claimed, already suffered too much, and the restraint and force required for feeding her against her will recapitulated her childhood trauma in a manner that violated empathy. In the language of futility, they argued that, "She stands no hope of achieving the things that she would value in her life. And shows no signs of revising these aspirations" (*Local Authority vs. E and Others* 2012).

One ED expert opined that treatment in a specialty EDs program could possibly improve Ms. E's condition and thus was ethically warranted. Relying on this advice, the official solicitor sought a forced-feeding order from the court on the grounds of best interests. E's case suggests that futility may not be clinically, legally, or ethically a coherent concept or compassionate approach when applied to SEEDs, so long as there is—as Judge Jackson emphasized—any reasonable chance of treatment response (*Local Authority vs. E and Others* 2012).

Betsi Cadwaladr University Local Health Board v. Miss W

In another case from the United Kingdom, *Betsi Cadwaladr University Local Health Board v. Miss W* (2016), Miss W, age 28, had been diagnosed with SEED for 20 years. She had been diagnosed with OCD at age 7 and AN at age 10. She had been admitted six times for inpatient treatment, amounting to a total of 10 years spent in inpatient care. Following a reduction in Miss W's weight, the Health Board raised two contrasting proposals for consideration. The first was for her to be re-fed under sedation, which would involve her being rendered unconscious for 6 months and fed via tube. The second was to discharge her to her parents' home with a community support program. This was predicated on the recognition that her condition was not treatable and acute treatment was no longer recommended.

Judge Jackson, the same jurist who heard Ms. E's case (*Local Authority vs. E and Others* 2012), also presided here. He heard testimony from Miss W as well as her treating psychiatrist, mother, and sister. He opined in his decision that, "After all that has happened, it now has to be accepted that it is beyond the power of doctors or family members, and certainly beyond the power of the court, to bring about an improvement in W's circumstances or an extension of her life." He ruled that Miss W's discharge to the community was the "least worst option" (*Betsi Cadwaladr University Local Health Board v. Miss W* 2016). Readmission to the hospital would not be part of the plan of care, even if her condition declined, unless her condition or circumstances were substantially altered. However, Judge Jackson approved the Health Board's proposal that, after a reasonable duration, if Miss W's cognition and symptoms suggested a willingness to move beyond her disorder, she should be reevaluated (*Betsi Cadwaladr University Local Health Board v. Miss W* 2016).

In this case, as in those of A.G. and S.A., one and the same judge made opposing rulings regarding patients with AN. In contrast to E's case, a medical consensus was found that further treatment for Miss W would cause harm without any real chance of benefit. This ruling is less definitive than that in A.G.'s case. Unlike the case of Ms. E, Judge Jackson declined to order treatment against Miss W's will yet agreed that she should be monitored and the decision revisited if Miss W became motivated to change.

NHS Foundation Trust v. Ms. X

Ms. X had struggled with AN for 14 years. She opposed forced feeding, even to save her life. She had been found to lack capacity to make decisions regarding ED treatment. The judge ruled that forced feeding against Ms. X's wishes was inhumane and violated her autonomy, opining that though nutrition could be compelled, psychological therapy could not (*NHS Foundation Trust v. Ms. X* 2014). This ruling did not consider emerging clinical research in three critical ways. First, research suggests that weight gain, even through forced feeding, significantly predicts survival. Second, the judge presumed psychotherapy could be beneficial but, because it is not effective if compelled, was not an option here. Research shows that without weight gain and improvement in ED symptoms, psychotherapy may enhance quality of life but not prognosis. Third, the possibility that weight gain may have a similar ameliorative effect on cognition and functional recovery, in terms of toleration of weight gain and psychological movement beyond preoccupation with food and weight, cannot be so handily dismissed. Weight restoration might have also restored Ms. X's capacity to voluntarily engage in and benefit from psychotherapy.

Recommendations and Conclusion

This chapter attempted to show that we must carefully assess each patient with SEEDs individually to determine what elements of active treatment are clinically and ethically suitable. At the same time, we should not deprive the small subset of seemingly "incurable" patients of the benefits of palliative care, ethical consultation, and equal access to good end-of-life care when deemed appropriate by experts in psychiatry, EDs, and medical ethics. Palliative care can and should be integrated into the care plan for those with serious illness along with treatments targeting cure and recovery. Palliative care has been shown to enhance the quality of life for patients with cancer, heart disease, and other life-limiting chronic conditions and has been credited with longer survival rates in some studies (Temel et al. 2010). Much less is known about the use of palliative care in psychiatric disorders. Given the high mortality rate in EDs compared with other psychiatric conditions, it seems appropriate to add palliative care to the treatment options for patients with SEEDs regardless of whether they forgo life-sustaining treatments. Although we hope that one day treatments as yet unknown may cure SEEDs, in the interim we are obligated to do our best to compassionately care for these patients who have suffered so deeply.

References

Betsi Cadwaladr University Local Health Board v Miss W (2016) EWCOP 13

Bosslet GT, Pope TM, Rubenfeld GD, et al: An official ATS/AACN/ACCP/ESICM/SCCM policy statement: responding to requests for potentially inappropriate treatments in intensive care units. Am J Respir Crit Care Med 191(11):1318–1330, 2015

Buzgova R, Sikorova L, Kozakova R, Jarosova D: Predictors of change in quality of life in patients with end-stage disease during hospitalization. J Palliat Care 32(2):69–76, 2017

Campbell AT, Aulisio MP: The stigma of "mental" illness: end stage anorexia and treatment refusal. Int J Eat Disord 45(5):627–634, 2012

Gans M, Gunn WB Jr: End stage anorexia: criteria for competence to refuse treatment. Int J Law Psychiatry 26(6):677–695, 2003

In the matter of A.G., New Jersey 2016

In the matter of S.A., New Jersey 2017

Local Authority v E and others, EWHC 1639, 2012

Lopez A, Yager J, Feinstein RE: Medical futility and psychiatry: palliative care and hospice care as a last resort in the treatment of refractory anorexia nervosa. Int J Eat Disord 43(4):372–377, 2010

NHS Foundation Trust v. Ms. X, EWCOP 35, 2014

Pies RW: Anorexia nervosa, "futility," and category errors. Am J Bioeth 15(7):44–46, 2015

Pope TM: Medical futility, in Guidance for Healthcare Ethics Committees. Edited by Hester DM, Schonfeld TL. Cambridge, UK, Cambridge University Press, 2012, pp 88–97

Reiser SJ, Dyck AJ, Curran W: Ethics in Medicine: Historical Perspectives and Contemporary Concerns. Cambridge, MA, MIT Press, 1977

Robinson P: Severe and Enduring Eating Disorder (SEED): Management of Complex Presentations of Anorexia and Bulimia Nervosa. Chichester, UK, Wiley, 2009

Robinson P, Kukucska R, Guidetti G, Leavey G: Severe and enduring anorexia nervosa (SEED-AN): a qualitative study of patients with 20+ years of anorexia nervosa. Eur Eat Disord Rev 23(4):318–326, 2015

Schneiderman L, Jecker NS, Jonsen AR: Medical futility: its meaning and implications. Ann Intern Med 112:949–954, 1990

Schreyer CC, Coughlin JW, Makhzoumi HG, et al: Perceived coercion in inpatients with anorexia nervosa: associations with illness severity and hospital course. Int J Eat Disord 49(4):407–412, 2016

Steinglass JE, Foerde K: Reward system abnormalities in anorexia nervosa: navigating a path forward. JAMA Psychiatry 75(10):993–994, 2018

Temel JS, Greer JA, Muzikansky A, et al: Early palliative care for patients with metastatic non-small-cell lung cancer. N Engl J Med 363(8):733–742, 2010

Touyz S, Hay P: Severe and enduring anorexia nervosa (SE-AN): in search of a new paradigm. J Eat Disord 3:26, 2015

Tripodoro VA, De Vito EL: What does end stage in neuromuscular diseases mean? Key approach-based transitions. Curr Opin Support Palliat Care 9(4):361–368, 2015

Westmoreland P, Johnson C, Stafford M, et al: Involuntary treatment of patients with life-threatening anorexia nervosa. J Am Acad Psychiatry Law 45(4):419–425, 2017

Yager J: Management of patients with chronic, intractable eating disorders, in Clinical Manual of Eating Disorders. Edited by Yager J, Powers PS. Washington, DC, American Psychiatric Publishing, 2007, pp 407–440

Yager J: The futility of arguing about medical futility in anorexia nervosa: the question is how would you handle highly specific circumstances? Am J Bioeth 15(7):47–50, 2015

12

Eating Disorders and Physician-Assisted Death

Mark Komrad, M.D.
Annette Hanson, M.D.

Physician-Assisted Death for Psychiatric Disorders

We use the term *physician-assisted death* (PAD) throughout this chapter to refer to both physician-assisted suicide, in which the patient ingests a lethal medication, and medical euthanasia, in which the lethal medication is administered by a physician or other health care provider, typically by injection. Although proponents of PAD object to use of the term *suicide* to refer to death by these means, we retain this nomenclature because it has been commonly accepted in both the medical and legal literature and avoids using language that discriminates between medical and psychiatric patients.

Many medical organizations consider PAD to be unethical, including the American Medical Association (1993), American Psychiatric Association (2016), American College of Physicians (Sulmasy and Muller 2017), and World Medical Association (2015). Nevertheless, physicians have occasionally deployed PAD "off the books" since the time of the ancient Greeks.

Only in recent years has the practice emerged as formally endorsed by several governments, supported as ethically acceptable by leading medical societies in those countries, and written into statutory law as permissible within certain guidelines.

The Benelux Experience

The first countries to open these gates via formal legislation were Belgium, The Netherlands, and Luxembourg, known collectively as the "Benelux" countries, all around 2002. In their respective legislations they allowed physicians to either directly administer legal injections (euthanasia) or provide prescriptions for patients to self-administer under certain circumstances (PAD). Patients must have conditions that are "unbearable." In The Netherlands, a key concept is *inveolbaar*, meaning that patients' suffering must be "palpable" to physicians (a criterion that is vulnerable to the dynamics of the doctor–patient dyad). Also, their condition must be deemed untreatable. The practice in Belgium has been similar to that in The Netherlands. However, further guidelines from the Belgian Order of Medicine were issued in 2019, specifically for the evaluation of psychiatric patients for euthanasia (Ordre des Medicines 2019). They suggested that two outside consultants be involved, at least one being a psychiatrist and one "specially qualified to judge the condition in question." Also, they recommended that, to be eligible, "the patient has had all possible evidenced-based treatments for the condition. When the psychiatric patient has exercised his right to refuse certain evidence-based treatments, the doctor cannot perform euthanasia." These guidelines are more stringent than both those in The Netherlands and those suggested for non-psychiatric patients in Belgium, but they are not changes to statutory laws. Prior to 2019, reports were published of euthanasia being allowed to proceed even when the consultants disagreed over the patient's eligibility and patients were allowed to refuse evidence-based treatments (Belgian Advisory Committee on Bioethics 2017; Thienpont et al. 2015).

The primary practice in Belgium and The Netherlands is euthanasia, or lethal injection by a physician. Assisted suicide by self-administered prescription barbiturates is more rare, although, unlike the United States, that self-administration must be overseen by a physician. The popularity of this option has grown at a remarkable pace. Now, nearly 4% of every human death in those countries occurs at the hand of a physician, typically pushing a syringe (La Commission Fédérale de Contrôle et d'Évaluation de l'Euthanasie 2018; Regional Euthanasia Review Committees 2018). Of particular significance is that the laws in Benelux countries removed from eligibility criteria any distinction between the conditions considered "terminal" and those not, as well as between "physical" and "mental" suffering

(Thienpont et al. 2015). This allowed individuals who were not terminally ill and whose suffering was predominantly mental or emotional to become potentially eligible. That opened the door to patients with psychiatric conditions, even those with no additional medical conditions, to receive death at the hands of a physician, often supported by the very treating psychiatrist who had previously been trying to prevent their suicide.

In The Netherlands, 311 patients with psychiatric disorders and predominantly "unbearable and untreatable mental suffering" had been euthanized through 2017. Their diagnoses ranged from schizophrenia and mood disorders to eating disorders (EDs) and borderline personality disorder. This excludes dementia, for which advance directives for euthanasia are legally accepted. Between 2015 and 2017, 310 people with dementia were euthanized in The Netherlands, some without advance directives (Regional Euthanasia Review Committees 2018).

In Belgium, 378 patients with psychiatric disorders had been euthanized through 2016. Lieve Thienpont, M.D., who has personally administered the largest percentage of these euthanasias, reported cases ranging from major mental illnesses to autistic spectrum disorders, fibromyalgia, complicated grief, PTSD, and personality disorder. Fifty percent of patients had a personality disorder diagnosis, most of which were borderline personality disorder (Nicolini et al. 2020; Thienpont et al. 2015).

The procession of practices and laws in these countries is a verifiable demonstration that a "slippery slope" phenomenon is not just a theoretical concern but a reality. In several high-profile examples, patients with tinnitus, gender dysphoria (unmitigated by several reassignment surgeries), blindness, alcoholism, and ego-dystonic homosexuality have been considered eligible and euthanized on request. The Dutch Voluntary Euthanasia Society, which has more than a quarter million members, has moved for the development of an over-the-counter suicide pill that would demedicalize the procedure altogether. In The Netherlands, leading politicians and government ministers are pushing to move beyond medical criteria to include "completed life" or "tired of living" as eligible thresholds for euthanasia. In Belgium, a convict serving a life sentence for rape claimed "unbearable mental suffering" due to his incarceration, and because there was no hope for amelioration of this suffering by parole, he was granted euthanasia by a review board. This permission was later withdrawn, however, when no physicians would perform the procedure (Reuters 2015). Remarkably, the Catholic Brothers of Charity, who run a large proportion of the psychiatric facilities in Belgium as their core mission and had been, not surprisingly, opposed to euthanasia for psychiatric patients heretofore, relented and decided to open their facilities to provide this "service" for eligible patients in April 2016, much to the displeasure of the Roman Curate (Camosy 2017).

The Canadian Experience

In 2016, at the instigation of its Supreme Court, the Canadian Parliament passed the C-14 Medical Aid in Dying (MAID) law, thus federally sanctioning euthanasia and assisted suicide nationally (*Carter v. Canada* 2015; Government of Canada 2016). Although the criteria resemble those in Benelux countries, the distinctions between physical and mental suffering have been maintained. Advocacy groups are pushing for expansion to mental disorders, but a large study group there has recommended that extreme caution be employed before extending MAID to individuals with psychiatric disorders (Council of Canadian Academies 2018). In addition, the C-14 statute has some unique language. It does not use *terminal illness* to characterize eligibility for euthanasia but instead refers to "death in the reasonably foreseeable future." However, that construct is undefined and vague and has been considered sufficient to justify some euthanasias for patients with life expectancies as long as 6 years. There were 2,704 deaths by euthanasia in Canada in 2017 alone, rising by 30% between the first and second halves of the year (Health Canada 2018). Moreover, in Ontario province, both changes in the ethics code of the College of Physicians and Surgeons of Ontario (2018) and a court ruling have declared it neither ethical nor legal for physicians, even if they object to the practice, to refuse to at least refer a patient for MAID to a physician comfortable with possibly approving or providing it.

The U.S. Experience

In the United States, legalization of PAD began in Oregon with adoption of the Death with Dignity Act in 1997 (Oregon Death with Dignity Act 1997). Using this law as a model, over the next 23 years, physician-assisted suicide was legalized in California, Colorado, District of Columbia, Hawaii, Vermont, and Washington. Montana maintained its criminal prohibition, but an appellate decision allowed patient consent as a defense to a charge of homicide against any participant (*Baxter v. State* 2009). Assisted suicide remains criminalized in all other states, despite repeated legislative efforts and court challenges by proponents. In 2017, 23 states rejected legalization bills and 2 states strengthened their criminal prohibitions (Hanson 2017).

Existing laws in the United States uniformly require that the patient's diagnosis and 6-month life expectancy be confirmed by two physicians. The patient must make two oral requests, separated by a minimum of 2 weeks, as well as a written request for lethal medication. If either physician suspects that the patient lacks medical decision-making capacity, the patient must be referred to a licensed psychiatrist or psychologist for a mental health evaluation. Despite this requirement, only about 5% of those given lethal prescriptions in Oregon received any psychiatric evaluation (Oregon Health Authority 2016). This low referral rate is concerning, given that as many as 26% of patients with a terminal illness requesting PAD in Oregon have co-existing clinical depression (Ganzini et al. 2008). Oregon's guide for health care professionals acknowledges that existing laws may not adequately protect patients with mental illness (Task Force to Improve the Care of Terminally-Ill Oregonians 2008).

Most of the data on the use of assisted suicide laws have been extracted from annual aggregate reports from Washington and Oregon, states with the most experience with PAD laws. Although PADs represent only a small proportion of annual mortality in each state, the rates of assisted death have risen exponentially every year. Most patients receiving lethal prescriptions are white, college educated, more than 65 years of age, and have cancer or chronic respiratory disease. However, prescriptions have also been given for an expanding list of conditions, such as diabetes, hepatitis, and alcoholic cirrhosis.

Unlike the Benelux countries, U.S. laws do not require that patients be suffering either physically or emotionally, only that they be terminally ill. However, common motivations for seeking PAD as seen in Oregon include concerns about the loss of autonomy and dignity and of the ability to enjoy usual activities, not current physical pain or suffering. These anxieties and fears are well known to mental health professionals, who have the skill set to address them, independent of particular psychiatric diagnoses. However, no requirements exist for attempted treatment with a mental health professional (Oregon Health Authority 2016).

American PAD laws explicitly prohibit the practice of euthanasia. They also do not require a witness attend the death or verify compliance with the law at the time of death. There has also been a movement to expand the use of PAD for patients with conditions such as dementia or Huntington's disease via use of an advance directive. This would require medical euthanasia for those who are too physically disabled to self-ingest medication or too cognitively impaired to understand the consequences of such procedures, even though they may be awake and alert (The Scrapbook 1999).

Eligibility for assisted suicide in the United States is based on the patient's prognosis, not diagnosis. There have been no cases of PAD primarily for mental illness, in the absence of physical illness. Yet this is likely to occur in states where PAD is legal, if a patient with a severe and persistent ED, for example, has a 6-month prognosis. (This assumes a way exists to conceive such a prognosis, because almost all medical complications of EDs are likely reversible with refeeding.) If such a prognosis could be enunciated, it would require participation of the patient's attending physician, a psychiatrist, and a second psychiatrist willing to confirm diagnosis, prognosis, and decision-making capacity. Because existing laws require the attending physician to write the prescription, a psychiatrist must also be trained and willing to order lethal medications.

Approved patients are prescribed a supply of lethal medication to take at a time and place of their own choosing. However, once released by the pharmacy, these patients have no protection from potential subtle and coercive influences by family and friends to ingest or refrain from ingesting the medication. Moreover, there is a risk that such a lethal supply of medication may be diverted for abuse or for suicide by some unapproved person. Current laws have no provision for tracking the location of the supply nor for recalling the medication if not used by a certain date.

Physician-Assisted Death for Eating Disorders

Thienpont et al. (2015) reported the clinical characteristics and outcomes for 100 consecutive requests for euthanasia in Belgium between 2007 and 2011. Ten of the requests were from people with EDs. One patient died of severe anorexia nervosa (AN) before being euthanized; the fate of the other nine patients was not described. The actual number of patients with EDs who are granted and die from PAD is likely to be significantly higher, given that it is estimated that almost half of all euthanasias in Belgium are not reported to the authorities (Smets et al. 2010). Because the reviewing commission closely protects clinical records, most of what is known about these cases is gleaned from media reports.

The most well-publicized case was that of a 44-year-old Belgian woman, Ann G., who sought treatment with a renowned ED specialist. She appeared on television to announce her intention to die but also accused her doctor of sexual abuse. Ultimately, her psychiatrist admitted the abuse, and his license was revoked, but by that time, another psychiatrist had approved Ann G.'s request for euthanasia, and she had already died. She cited bitterness over her abuse as one reason she wanted to die (Cook 2013; Fiano-Chesser 2013).

Another sexual abuse victim, an unnamed young woman in her twenties, was euthanized in The Netherlands due to AN as well as multiple other diagnoses: PTSD, chronic depression, and obsessions and compulsions. She had a history of self-harming behavior and had been known to hallucinate, according to the Dutch Euthanasia Commission, which released a clinical summary to the media following criticism of the death and increasing public scrutiny of the practice (Doughty 2016).

In 2018, the story of 29-year-old Aurelia Brouwers was featured in a television documentary and the front-page story of a regional newspaper. Diagnosed with severe anxiety, depression, ED, and psychosis, Brouwers had attempted suicide, had self-harmed several times in the past, and had a prior 3-year psychiatric admission. When her own psychiatrists disagreed about her eligibility for PAD, she contacted the Levenseindekliniek (End of Life Clinic) in The Hague, a clinic known to approve individuals who had been denied elsewhere. She announced her death on Facebook, with the hope of inspiring other people with mental illness to consider this "treatment." She was even filmed by the media visiting a funeral home to prepare the ceremonies to follow her death (Sherwood 2018).

Noa Pothoven, a 17-year-old Dutch teenager with a history of sexual assaults, PTSD, and severe AN, applied to the Levenseindekliniek for euthanasia in 2018. Her request was refused. However, her family, with the support of her physicians, stood by as Pothoven voluntarily stopped eating and drinking in 2019. She was not involuntarily hospitalized and died at home (Brown 2019). Although this case was falsely reported at first in the media as a euthanasia (because of her previous unsuccessful application), it raised international awareness of euthanasia practices in The Netherlands for psychiatric patients in general and patients with AN in particular. However, the world believed the misreported story and accelerated its spread, precisely because of its plausibility, because euthanasia for AN does indeed happen in Benelux countries. Moreover, that such a young woman would not be vigorously treated but instead be allowed to die may reflect a change in the conceptualization of the treatability of psychiatric disorders in a society that has shifted its approach to such disorders, thanks to the practice of psychiatric euthanasia for 17 years in The Netherlands. After that country statutorily defined a domain of cases that are "untreatable" and "unbearable" (and thus eligible for euthanasia) in 2002, with advanced medical disease as the original paradigm, that silo gradually became populated with psychiatric cases. This appears to have led that society, and even its psychiatric profession, to move the fulcrum on which distinctions between hopeful and unhopeful cases balance. Cases like that of 17-year-old Pothoven might previously have been considered still treatable, but thanks to psychiatric euthanasia becoming normative, such cases may have become reconceived as untreatable and thus eligible for compassionate "termination" by withdrawing treatment, even if ineligible for euthanasia per se.

These cases illustrate the clinical complexity of patients seeking PAD on the basis of an ED. When assessing prognosis and incurability, which condition should this opinion be based on: the ED, mood disorder, personality disorder, or trauma-induced condition? Moreover, evidence has shown that patients with severe and enduring AN can make significant additional progress if given more specialized treatment (Calugi et al. 2017). Lack of access geographically or financially to such advanced treatment centers makes the concept of futility fraught with considerable complexity and lack of clarity (see Chapter 11). So, whether working with a statutory paradigm of a "terminal" or an "untreatable" illness as a condition for PAD, this kind of uncertainty about prognosis and treatability make EDs particularly difficult to reckon with, even by the most permissive European practices.

Concerns About Capacity

As discussed in Chapter 4, patients' capacity, or lack thereof, is a threshold question that must be addressed. Similarly, all PAD laws require an assessment of medical decision-making capacity, although the assessment may be made by a physician who is not necessarily trained or experienced in ED treatment. None of the jurisdictions in the United States requires that either the first or second opinions for PAD be provided by a specialist in a patient's particular "terminal" disorder, nor are either of the two evaluating physicians required to have any specific training or experience with doing capacity evaluations.

Capacity is a dimensional phenomenon, but determining the threshold for consent capacity has heretofore been applied by clinicians in situations in which patients asked to withdraw life-sustaining care. It was not a death administered or provided by a physician for the purpose of causing death, as in PAD. No criteria have been developed for determining capacity for PAD in which the physician is literally asked to kill a patient or offer patients the means to kill themselves.

The motivated behavior to starve in an ED is clearly epiphenomenal, indeed definitional, to the condition itself. That morbid choice, independent of explicit suicidality, can result in death. Would a clinician's threshold for determining a patient's capacity is sufficient for PAD be different if the patient's goal is simply to not eat, compared with the goal of explicitly wanting to die? Moreover, the drive to eschew eating, as well as the impairment in cognitive flexibility and insight caused by extreme weight loss, are manifest impairments in the capacity to evince a truly autonomous decision, free from the distorted drives and desires of the illness itself (Konstantakopoulos et al. 2011). Thus, patients with EDs have some degree of diminished capacity, and however subtle that diminishment might be, it is an obstacle to proving that they have an ethically appropriate level of autonomy to give informed consent for the irreversible and certain decision to die by PAD. This creates a situation in which the person with an ED would require *proxy* consent for PAD. Currently, no country allows PAD by proxy consent, although in 2010, more than 1,000 people in Belgium were euthanized without either advance or direct consent (Chambaere et al. 2010).

In addition to the direct effects of the illness itself, capacity evaluation involves assessment of contextual factors such as social support, financial resources, and access to specialty services. No psychometric tools or measures exist to guide clinicians in this particular assessment, nor are any clinical or legal standards established for the competence to request PAD. A faulty or poorly performed capacity assessment cannot be challenged in court, nor can a lethal prescription be withdrawn if inadvertently given to a patient who lacks capacity. This is a particularly concerning aspect of PAD laws, because there is no provision for the concept of "fluid" capacity, or loss of capacity, as the disease advances. Because a competent decision must be made freely and voluntarily, a request for PAD must also necessarily involve an assessment of "noncoercion," a concept not typically part of assessing medical decision-making capacity but statutorily required by existing U.S. laws. People with AN may experience coercion by family members when faced with involuntary treatment, and caregiver exhaustion could potentially be a coercive factor in requests for PAD (Ishay 1989). Psychiatrists who routinely assess capacity generally accept that high-risk medical interventions require a more intense level of scrutiny. The decision to request death would certainly meet this standard (Charland et al. 2016).

Ethical Cautionary Notes

Since the original Hippocratic Oath and its covenantal value at the heart of medicine—"I shall give no man a poison nor advise another to do so"—the field has professed a set of values. Edmund Pellegrino noted that such shared and publicly professed values are "the magnetic core that can help to create a moral community, creating a sense of collective responsibility for a profession" (American Association for Advancement of Science 2020). Medicine has articulated for several millennia its fundamental ethos to care and comfort but not kill. Physicians have long been able to stand aside in a posture of compassionate attendance on a suffering patient (compassion, literally meaning "to suffer with"). Psychiatrists in particular have a skill set and purpose, independent of diagnosis—what Scott Kim and Willem Lemmens called "a core imperative…compassionately and skillfully helping patients, even through periods of sustained suffering during which people lose the will to live" (Kim and Lemmens 2016, p. E338). Psychiatrists prevent suicide, they do not provide it. John Maher, editor-in-chief of the *Journal of Ethics in Mental Health*, asserted that, "Just as the Pope should not perform abortions, and the Dalai Lama should not take up arms, a psychiatrist should not counsel or abet suicide, for in doing so [they] have misunderstood and betrayed [their] vocation and profession" (Maher 2017, p. 4).

The burden of caring for patients with chronic and difficult conditions, such as EDs, on professionals and caregivers lures us into projectively identifying with the patients' hopelessness and helplessness. As Paul McHugh warned during the time of Kevorkian, psychiatrists can inadvertently collude with this helplessness, even though we, of all physicians, should know better:

> Patients are seduced…by isolating them, sustaining their despair, revoking alternatives, stressing examples of others choosing to die, and sweetening the deadly poison by speaking of death with dignity. If even psychiatrists succumb to this complicity with death, what can be expected of the lay public? (McHugh 2006, p. 80)

Who would be appropriate witnesses for a patient with ED to consent to suicide by self-administered medication or to death by euthanasia? The profound effect of ordinary suicide on loved ones, friends, and even a community of strangers is well documented (Cerel et al. 2019). For physicians themselves, the emotional trauma of evaluating for or administering PAD is well described, even for those who merely refer the patient to a colleague willing to consider evaluating or providing it (Stevens 2006).

Recommendations for Clinicians Who Are Asked to Evaluate a Patient Considering PAD

Outside the Benelux countries, the role of psychiatrists in PAD is typically limited to being asked to consult on the case of a patient seeking PAD. This is usually either in one of the U.S. states where it is legal or in Canada, although psychiatrists are beginning to be approached to evaluate and "sign off" on patients who hope to go abroad for PAD, typically to Switzerland, which currently has a system available for this kind of "medical tourism." How might a psychiatrist respond to such consultative requests?

Even though a psychiatrist may not ultimately be writing a lethal prescription or administering the injection, participation in the evaluation process equals participation in the chain of medical authority. This chain may ultimately lead to a physician actively causing a patient's death by providing a means of killing and not merely providing comfort while a natural death occurs. This is not palliative care. Moral culpability must be considered and measured, not only against one's personal values but also against the professed values to which the psychiatrist has sworn. Much like a sworn police officer, entry into the profession of medicine signifies commitment to an ethos that transcends personal values. As noted, some of the most important world bodies that keep vigilance over those professed values in medicine have clear objections to these practices. Recent attempts have been made to soften the stances of the American Medical Association and the World Medical Association, which assert that assisted suicide and medical euthanasia are unethical. However, as of this writing, both organizations have withstood these efforts and maintain firm positions that reflect the Hippocratic legacy (Frieden 2019; Komrad 2018). Similarly, regarding participation in a chain of culpability, if not the final moral act, both organization assert that it is unethical to participate in executions, and the American Psychiatric Association proscribes psychiatrists' participation in torture interrogations (American Medical Association 2016; American Psychiatric Association 2014; Komrad et al. 2018; World Medical Association 2018).

When fulfilling a request to psychiatrically evaluate a patient for PAD, whether for capacity or to rule out a treatable psychiatric disorder, psychiatrists should exercise extreme caution about entering the chain of moral culpability for the outcome, even if they are legally immune. However, it would certainly be within the scope, mission, and core ethos of psychiatry to perform this evaluation for our standard intentions: to identify tools in our arsenal of skills that will help patients' suffering, fortify their defenses, shore up their support systems, be present to their suffering, provide and advocate for access to state-of-the-art treatment, and even help make meaning of suffering that cannot be entirely lysed. Proffering such services to patients referred to us for evaluation for PAD deploys the most effective powers of our specialty in a manner that is ethically congruent with more than 2,000 years of developed medical ethics, not just dutifully, but virtuously.

References

American Association for Advancement of Science: Should There be An Oath for Scientists and Engineers? Washington, DC, American Association for Advancement of Science, 2020. Available at: https://www.aaas.org/programs/scientific-responsibility-human-rights-law/should-there-be-oath-scientists-and-engineers. Accessed July 25, 2020.

American Medical Association: Code of Medical Ethics Opinion 5.7: Physician-Assisted Suicide. Chicago, IL, American Medical Association, 1993. Available at: https://www.ama-assn.org/delivering-care/ethics/physician-assisted-suicide. Accessed January 12, 2019.

American Medical Association: Code of Medical Ethics Opinion 9.7.3: Capital Punishment. Chicago, IL, American Medical Association, 2016. Available at: https://www.ama-assn.org/delivering-care/ethics/capital-punishment. Accessed January 12, 2019.

American Psychiatric Association: Position Statement on Psychiatric Participation in Interrogation of Detainees. Arlington, VA, American Psychiatric Association, 2014. Available at: https://www.psychiatry.org/File%20Library/About-APA/Organization-Documents-Policies/Policies/Position-2014-Interrogation-Detainees-Psychiatric-Participation.pdf. Accessed January 12, 2019.

American Psychiatric Association: Position Statement on Medical Euthanasia. Arlington, VA, American Psychiatric Association, 2016. Available at: https://www.psychiatry.org/File%20Library/About-APA/Organization-Documents-Policies/Policies/Position-2016-Medical-Euthanasia.pdf. Accessed January 12, 2019.

Baxter v. State, 224 P.3d 1211 (2009)

Belgian Advisory Committee on Bioethics: Opinion No. 73 of 11 September 2017 on Euthanasia in Case of Non-Terminally Ill Patients, Psychological Suffering and Psychiatric Disorders. Brussels, Belgium, 2017. Available at: https://www.health.belgium.be/sites/default/files/uploads/fields/fpshealth_theme_file/opinion_73_web.pdf. Accessed January 12, 2019.

Brown E: 17 year old rape victim Noa Pothoven ends her life (but it wasn't state sanctioned euthanasia). DutchReview.com, June 5, 2019. Available at: https://dutchreview.com/news/international/noa-pothoven-ends-her-life-but-it-wasnt-euthanasia. Accessed June 5, 2019.

Calugi S, Ghoch M, Grave R: Intensive enhanced cognitive behavioural therapy for severe and enduring anorexia nervosa. Behav Res Ther 89:41–48, 2017

Camosy C: Euthanasia and the Belgian Brothers of Charity. First Things, September 26, 2017. Available at: https://www.firstthings.com/web-exclusives/2017/09/euthanasia-and-the-belgian-brothers-of-charity. Accessed January 12, 2019.

Carter v. Canada, 2015 SCC 5 (2015)

Cerel J, Brown M, Maple M, et al: How many people are exposed to suicide? Not six. Suicide Life Threat Behav 49(2):529–534, 2019

Chambaere K, Bilsen J, Cohen J, et al: Physician-assisted deaths under the euthanasia law in Belgium: a population-based survey. CMAJ 182:895–901, 2010

Charland L, Lemmens T, Wada K: Decision-making capacity to consent to medical assistance in dying for persons with mental disorders. Journal of Ethics in Mental Health, May 25, 2016. Available at: https://jemh.ca/issues/v9/documents/JEMH_Open-Volume_Benchmark_Decision_Making_to_Consent_to_Medical_Assistance_in_Dying-May2016-rev.pdf. Accessed January 12, 2019.

College of Physicians and Surgeons of Ontario: Medical Assistance in Dying (website) updated December 2018. Available at: https://www.cpso.on.ca/Physicians/Policies-Guidance/Policies/Medical-Assistance-in-Dying. Accessed January 12, 2019.

La Commission Fédérale de Contrôle et d'Évaluation de l'Euthanasie: CFCEE Rapport Euthanasie 2018: 8e Rapport aux Chambres Législatives: Chiffres des Années 2016–2017. Brussels, Belgium, CFCEE, 2018. Available at: https://organesdeconcertation.sante.belgique.be/fr/documents/cfcee-rapport-euthanasie-2018. Unofficial English translation available at: https://www.dyingforchoice.com/docs/Belgium_Annual_Report_2016-2017_En.pdf. Accessed January 12, 2019.

Cook M: Another speed bump for Belgian euthanasia. BioEdge, February 8, 2013. Available at: https://www.bioedge.org/bioethics/another_speed_bump_for_belgian_ euthanasia/10388. Accessed January 12, 2019.

Council of Canadian Academies: The State of Knowledge on Medical Assistance in Dying Where a Mental Disorder Is the Sole Underlying Medical Condition. Ottawa, ON, Council of Canadian Academies, 2018c. Available at: https://cca-reports.ca/wp-content/uploads/2018/12/The-State-of-Knowledge-on-Medical-Assistance-in-Dying-Where-a-Mental-Disorder-is-the-Sole-Underlying-Medical-Condition.pdf. Accessed January 12, 2019.

Doughty S: Sex abuse victim in her 20s allowed to choose euthanasia. Mail Online, May 10, 2016. Available at: https://www.dailymail.co.uk/news/article-3583783/Sex-abuse-victim-20s-allowed-choose-euthanasia-Holland-doctors-decided-post-traumatic-stress-conditions-uncurable.html. Accessed January 12, 2019.

Fiano-Chesser C: Belgian woman suffering from anorexia euthanized. Live Action News, February 13, 2013. Available at: https://www.liveaction.org/news/belgian-woman-suffering-from-anorexia-euthanized. Accessed January 12, 2019.

Frieden J: Physician assisted suicide once again divides AMA members. Med Page Today, June 12, 2019. Available at: https://www.medpagetoday.com/meetingcoverage/ama/80384. Accessed June 13, 2019.

Ganzini L, Goy E, Dobscha S: Prevalence of depression and anxiety in patients requesting physicians' aid in dying. BMJ 337:a1682, 2008

Government of Canada: Legislative background: medical assistance in dying (Bill C-14). Ottawa, ON, Government of Canada, 2016. Available at: https://www.justice.gc.ca/eng/rp-pr/other-autre/ad-am/ad-am.pdf. Accessed January 12, 2019

Hanson J: A momentum shift against assisted suicide. Washington Examiner, September 3, 2017. Available at: https://www.washingtonexaminer.com/a-momentum-shift-against-assisted-suicide. Accessed January 12, 2019.

Health Canada: Third Interim Report on Medical Assistance in Dying in Canada. Ottawa, ON, Health Canada, 2018. Available at: https://www.canada.ca/content/dam/hc-sc/documents/services/publications/health-system-services/medical-assistance-dying-interim-report-june-2018/medical-assistance-dying-interim-report-june-2018-eng.pdf. Accessed January 12, 2019.

Ishay R: Euthanasia: the slippery slope. WMJ 36:44–45, 1989

Kim S, Lemmens T: Should assisted dying be legalized in Canada? CMAJ 188:E337–E339, 2016

Komrad M: Euthanasia vs. plagiarism: a strange international drama. Psychiatric Times, October 10, 2018. Available at: https://www.psychiatrictimes.com/couch-crisis/euthanasia-versus-plagiarism-strange-international-drama. Accessed June 13, 2018.

Komrad M, Pies R, Hanson A, Geppert C: Assessing competency for physician-assisted suicide is unethical. J Clin Psychiatry 79(6), 2018

Konstantakopoulos G, Tchanturia K, Surguladze S, David A: Insight in eating disorders: clinical and cognitive correlates. Psychol Med 41:1951–1961, 2011

Maher J: What troubles me as a psychiatrist about the physician assisted suicide debate in Canada. Journal of Ethics in Mental Health. Open Volume 10:1–5, 2017. Available at: https://jemh.ca/issues/open/documents/JEMH%20vol%2010%20editorial.pdf. Accessed January 12, 2019.

McHugh P: The Mind Has Mountains: Reflections on Society and Psychiatry. Baltimore, MD, Johns Hopkins University Press, 2006

Nicolini M, Peteet J, Donovan K, Kim S: Euthanasia and assisted suicide of persons with psychiatric disorders: the challenge of personality disorders. Psychol Med 50(4):575–582, 2020

Ordre des Medicines: Deontological Guidelines for the Application of Euthanasia in Patients Who Suffer Psychologically as a Result of a Psychiatric Disorder. Brussels, Belgium, Ordre des Medicines, 2019. Available at: https://www.ordomedic.be/nl/adviezen/advies/deontologische-richtlijnen-voor-de-toepassing-van-euthanasie-bij-patienten-die-psychisch-lijden-ten-gevolge-van-een-psychiatrische-aandoening. Accessed July 25, 2020.

Oregon Death With Dignity Act, ORS §§ 127.800–127.897 (1997)

Oregon Health Authority: Oregon Death With Dignity Act: Data Summary, June 2016. Available at: https://www.oregon.gov/oha/ph/providerpartnerresources/evaluationresearch/deathwithdignityact/documents/year19.pdf. Accessed January 12, 2019.

Regional Euthanasia Review Committees: Annual Report 2017. The Hague, The Netherlands, 2018. Available at: https://english.euthanasiecommissie.nl/binaries/euthanasiecommissie-en/documents/publications/annual-reports/2002/annual-reports/annual-reports/RTE_annual+report+2017.pdf. Accessed January 12, 2019.

Reuters: Doctors block Belgian murderer's euthanasia. World News, January 6, 2015. Available at: https://www.reuters.com/article/us-belgium-euthanasia-prisoner/doctors-block-belgian-murderers-euthanasia-idUSKBN0KF1HA20150106. Accessed January 12, 2019.

The Scrapbook: The slope is slippery. The Weekly Standard, March 29, 1999. Available at: https://www.weeklystandard.com/the-scrapbook/the-slope-is-slippery. Accessed January 12, 1999.

Sherwood H: A woman's final Facebook message before euthanasia: "I'm ready for my trip now…." The Guardian, March 17, 2018. Available at: https://www.theguardian.com/society/2018/mar/17/assisted-dying-euthanasia-netherlands. Accessed January 12, 2019.

Smets T, Bilsen J, Cohen J, et al: Reporting of euthanasia in medical practice in Flanders, Belgium: cross sectional analysis of reported and unreported cases. BMJ 341:c5174, 2010

Stevens K: Emotional and psychological effects of physician-assisted suicide and euthanasia on participating physicians. Issues Law Med 21(3):187–200, 2006

Sulmasy L, Muller P: Ethics and the legalization of physician-assisted suicide: an American College of Physicians position paper. Ann Intern Med 167:576–578, 2017

Task Force to Improve the Care of Terminally-Ill Oregonians: The Oregon Death With Dignity Act: A Guidebook for Healthcare Professionals, 2nd Edition. Portland, OR, Center for Ethics in Health Care, Oregon Health Sciences University, 2008

Thienpont L, Verhofstadt M, Van Loon T, et al: Euthanasia requests, procedures and outcomes for 100 Belgian patients suffering from psychiatric disorders: a retrospective, descriptive study. BMJ Open 5:e007454, 2015

World Medical Association: Resolution on Euthanasia. Ferney-Voltaire, France, World Medical Association, April 2015. Available at: https://www.wma.net/policies-post/wma-declaration-on-euthanasia. Accessed January 12, 2019.

World Medical Association: WMA Resolution on Prohibition of Physician Participation in Capital Punishment. Ferney-Voltaire, France, World Medical Association, 2018. Available at: https://www.wma.net/policies-post/wma-resolution-on-prohibition-of-physician-participation-in-capital-punishment. Accessed January 12, 2019.

Index

Page numbers printed in **boldface** type refer to tables.